P9-DTS-945

Clark Library
University of Portland

Clark Library
University of Portland

PROMISING CARE

PROMISING CARE

How We Can Rescue Health Care by Improving It

Donald M. Berwick

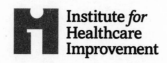

Institute *for* Healthcare Improvement

JB JOSSEY-BASS™
A Wiley Brand

b13804376
i9

RA
399
.A3
B48
2014

·i 14283694

862041347

Cover design by JPuda
Cover image: (abstract) © Ralf Hiemisch/Getty; (tree) © Martin Ruegner/Getty
Copyright © 2014 by Donald M. Berwick. All rights reserved.

Published by Jossey-Bass
A Wiley Brand
One Montgomery Street, Suite 1200, San Francisco, CA 94104-4594
www.josseybass.com

No part of this publication may be reproduced, stored in a retrieval system, or
transmitted in any form or by any means, electronic, mechanical, photocopying,
recording, scanning, or otherwise, except as permitted under Section 107 or 108 of the
1976 United States Copyright Act, without either the prior written permission of the
publisher, or authorization through payment of the appropriate per-copy fee to the
Copyright Clearance Center, Inc., 222 Rosewood Drive, Danvers, MA 01923,
978-750-8400, fax 978-646-8600, or on the Web at www.copyright.com. Requests
to the publisher for permission should be addressed to the Permissions Department,
John Wiley & Sons, Inc., 111 River Street, Hoboken, NJ 07030, 201-748-6011,
fax 201-748-6008, or online at www.wiley.com/go/permissions.

Limit of Liability/Disclaimer of Warranty: While the publisher and author have used
their best efforts in preparing this book, they make no representations or warranties
with respect to the accuracy or completeness of the contents of this book and specifically
disclaim any implied warranties of merchantability or fitness for a particular purpose.
No warranty may be created or extended by sales representatives or written sales
materials. The advice and strategies contained herein may not be suitable for your
situation. You should consult with a professional where appropriate. Neither the
publisher nor author shall be liable for any loss of profit or any other commercial
damages, including but not limited to special, incidental, consequential, or other
damages. Readers should be aware that Internet Web sites offered as citations and/or
sources for further information may have changed or disappeared between the time this
was written and when it is read.

Jossey-Bass books and products are available through most bookstores. To contact
Jossey-Bass directly call our Customer Care Department within the U.S.
at 800-956-7739, outside the U.S. at 317-572-3986, or fax 317-572-4002.

Wiley publishes in a variety of print and electronic formats and by print-on-demand.
Some material included with standard print versions of this book may not be included in
e-books or in print-on-demand. If this book refers to media such as a CD or DVD that
is not included in the version you purchased, you may download this material at
http://booksupport.wiley.com. For more information about Wiley products, visit
www.wiley.com.

Library of Congress Cataloging-in-Publication Data has been applied for and is on file at
the Library of Congress.

ISBN 978-1-118-79588-0 (cloth) — ISBN 978-1-118-79585-9 (pdf) —
ISBN 978-1-118-79583-5 (epub)

Printed in the United States of America
FIRST EDITION
HB Printing   10 9 8 7 6 5 4 3 2 1

CONTENTS

To Howard H. Hiatt, MD—my mentor, friend, and model. For decades of gracious help, warm counsel, and constant encouragement.

As this book was nearing its final stages, we lost our colleague, friend, and editor, Andy Pasternack. Andy was, for over two decades, a generous and encouraging champion of our writing and of the health care improvement work that is the subject of this book. His optimism and energy fueled and guided us. We are deeply grateful to have had him with us on our journey. He made us better, and we miss him.

—Don Berwick

PREFACE

IF I HAD known in advance how important serendipity would be in shaping the arc of my career in health care improvement, I would have been very worried. Could so much, indeed, be left to pure chance?

But, there you have it. If it had not been raining on the night that I met a stranger named Paul Batalden at a dinner meeting, I would not have offered him a ride to his Boston hotel, and he would not have had a chance to tell me how important it was that I learn about W. Edwards Deming, whose name I had not known.

If I had not on a moment's impulse decided to cold-call AT&T Bell Laboratories and ask the switchboard who was in charge of quality there, Blan Godfrey would not have had the chance to answer his phone and invite me down there and, in a few short weeks, to become one of my most valued friends and mentors. Without Blan, there would have been no National Demonstration Project on Quality Improvement in Health Care (NDP); it was his idea. And without the NDP, there would have never been an Institute for Healthcare Improvement (IHI).

And if Dick Sharpe had not been assigned to Blan and me as our John A. Hartford Foundation Project Officer for the NDP, he would never have had the chance to suggest three years later that the NDP was promising enough that a new, nonprofit organization should be built upon its foundation—the idea that became the IHI.

If my father, and, after that, my wife, had not become seriously ill, I would never have had to confront the searing emotions that drove me into the arms of the patient-centeredness and patient safety movement (as I explained in my speeches "Quality Comes Home" and "Escape Fire") from the inside—my experience—rather than from the outside—my intellect—emotions that, absolutely literally, turned my hair white.

The happenstance continues. It propelled my colleagues and me through the ten years punctuated by the eleven speeches collected in the book *Escape Fire*, which was "Volume One" of the collected IHI National Forum speeches from 1992 to 2002, and it equally propels the journey of sixteen more speeches now collected here, in "Volume Two," *Promising Care*, which comprises talks from 2003 through 2012. This volume differs from *Escape Fire* in that it includes a few speeches that were not delivered at an IHI National Forum, such as "The Epitaph of Profession," which was my John Hunt Lecture at the Royal College of General Practice in England, my address to my daughter's graduating Yale School of Medicine class, and "To Isaiah," which I delivered as the 2012 Harvard Medical School and Harvard School of Dental Medicine Class Day speaker.

As the speeches in *Promising Care* click by in my mind, I can once again see serendipity at work, as my thinking evolved through the first decade of the twenty-first century. Dozens of transitions occur to me, but I discern five of particular power to shape my views.

First was the arrival of "spread" and "scale" at the center of my aims.

For the first decade and a half of my improvement work, I was satisfied, if not entirely content, to help encourage prototypes of success. The National Demonstration Project was aptly named; the goal was proof of concept, and "demonstration" was, we thought, adequate; the mainstream would follow along. We were wrong. We had underestimated the depth of the taproots of the status quo, and we did not at first understand that bringing good change to full scale needed to become an enterprise of its own. From about 2000 to 2005, IHI, and I, took on large-scale change with passion. The serendipity there had several forms. It just so happened that my second son, Dan, had been working on political campaigns for several years, and it just so happened that I asked him on a car ride how expert political campaigners thought about scale. His answer was complex and eloquent, but one line especially stuck with me: "Some is not a number, soon is not a time." And from that idea was born the IHI's 100,000 Lives Campaign, and eventually its successor, the 5 Million Lives Campaign. One conversation; six years of work.

And, it just so happened that a college roommate of Ben's (my other son) named Joe McCannon walked into the doors of IHI looking for a job just about then. Joe's fertile mind and inconceivable level of energy brought the Campaigns into reality, and, I believe, changed history with respect to how we think today about large-scale spread.

Second was my new conceptualization of "patient-centeredness" as a foundation for improvement.

At the time of *Escape Fire*, I would not have written "foundation" in that sentence; I would have said, "component." It took years of gentle prodding from scholars who knew it first—Maureen Bisognano, Susan Edgman-Levitan, and Bev Johnson, for example—and one unwelcome, serious illness in a loved one, for me rather suddenly to realize one day with a healthy dose of anger that authentic patient-centeredness (better, "person-centeredness") is not an *element* of an agenda for improvement; it is a *precondition* of improvement. I collected those notions in my speech to the American Board of Internal Medicine Foundation, "The True Nature of Patient-Centered Care: Confessions of an Extremist." The unexpected email that I received one day from Mrs. Jackie Gruzenski nailed down that idea for me irrevocably and shaped my Yale School of Medicine graduation speech.

A third twist (harder to pin down its accidental source) was my realization, as the first decade of the twenty-first century closed, that we simply could not tolerate a separation between what Brent James calls "care outcomes" and "cost outcomes."

As a student of Deming's, I knew from the late 1980s on that we in health care ought generally to "adopt the new philosophy." That phrase was one of Deming's famous "14 Points for Top Leaders," explicated in his book *Out of the Crisis*. "The new philosophy" was to realize that better quality was the keystone to sustainable economies and jobs, with lower total cost as the link. We in the health care quality movement, and health care overall, had not made that link; indeed, we had no sound conception at all of "total cost," nor, to judge us by results, do we yet get it. And I came to realize as the decade wore on, even before the Great Recession, and urgently after it, that if we do not find the discipline to use what we had learned about improvement to reduce costs, the loss will be incalculable. John Whittington and Tom Nolan had elegantly rung that bell with their framing of the "Triple Aim": better care for individuals, better health for populations, and lower per capita cost, and the Triple Aim soon became a mainstay of my lectures. It has since swept the world at a pace and scale that no other IHI contribution rivals.

The new philosophy acquired precision with the arrival of "Lean thinking" and "Lean production" full force in health care. I had been acquainted with this powerful framing ever since my (chance) encounter with the MIT project, "The Future of the Automobile," and my tutoring by one of its genius scholars, Jim Womack. But it was the enthusiasm of expert practitioners like Patty Gabow, John Toussaint, and Gary Kaplan, and the generous, brilliant help of my accidental new friend, Amory Lovins, that gave me an entirely new and durable understanding of the nature of abundance itself. From that time onward, cost has been for me a dimension of quality, period.

Fourth, pure chance brought me, with utter surprise, to the interface between the quality movement and the world of politics.

Inklings came in the IHI National Forum plenary addresses by Gloria Steinem and, later, Paul O'Neill, which hinted at the power of political

influences on improvement and of the potential for mobilization of interest groups for improvement. But who could have known that, the day
after Christmas 2008, I would get a call from Senator Tom Daschle, then
the probable nominee for Health and Human Services Secretary, asking
me if I would consider taking a job in the new administration of Barack
Obama as administrator of the Centers for Medicare & Medicaid Services. It took a while—eighteen months to be exact—before the winds
of Washington would carry me into that job as a "recess appointee" for
the next seventeen months, reporting not to Senator Daschle but to Secretary Kathleen Sebelius, but it was a life-changing, mind-changing
happenstance. Indelibly, that experience taught me the need for and the
power of political work to permit improvement to thrive. It changed how
I think and how I act, and the speeches herein from the time that followed that service—"The Moral Test" and "To Isaiah"—mark that
change. The personal experience of illness that led me to write "Escape
Fire" in 1999 radicalized my passion for improvement; the personal
experience of Washington radicalized my view of the role of power in
protecting the vulnerable and the future. I can never go back.

Fifth, chance favored a mental turn for me that is still in its early stages
but is foreshadowed in this volume.

It is an awkward turn, because I do not yet fully comprehend it, nor
is it particularly consistent with my style and theory to date. To give it
a name, let's call it "spirituality," or, in a common term of the day,
"mindfulness."

I owe this turn to chance encounters again, this time to stumbling
upon some new mentors, including Jon Kabat-Zinn, Richie Davidson,
David Kindig, and Wayne Jonas. I have known for some time that our
normal view of health care and health is much too confining. It is mini-
malist, and not fully in accord with the World Health Organization's very
definition of health: "Health is a state of complete physical, mental and
social well-being and not merely the absence of disease or infirmity." The
words for the future are, I think, ones like Kaiser Permanente's slogan:
"Thrive"; Wayne Jonas's term: "flourishing"; and Jon Kabat-Zinn's:
"mindfulness" and "lovingkindness." These thoughts seep into my latest
speeches, most directly in the speech called, "Squirrel," which, if I must
choose, I probably would select as my favorite of this collection, especially when it asks, "What do you want? What do you really want? What
do you really, really want?" I have never met a more powerful sequence
of questions in three decades of search for the keys to improvement.

Indeed, if my work ever sees a third volume of collected speeches ten
or twelve more years ahead, I will not be surprised if the search for

mindfulness, presence, and deep-founded generosity prove to be at their collective core, much as process-mindedness infused *Escape Fire*, and the hope for large-scale change runs as a vein through the speeches in *Promising Care*.

So, kind reader, I hope that you enjoy reading these talks, as I enjoyed writing them. But, do not hope that you will find herein a clearly mapped and fully preconceived story unfolding, a structure brick upon brick. You won't. That is not how my career or my thinking has evolved. Accidents good and bad have punctuated the flow every step of the way, about which perhaps the best that can be said, what I *hope* can be said, is this: "He learned."

Acknowledgments

I offer deep thanks to my IHI colleagues Jane Roessner, Val Weber, and Dan Schummers for their skill and entrepreneurship in guiding this project in a breathtakingly short time, and to Markus Josephson for helping to keep it on track. Each of the commenters whom we asked for brief introductory essays delivered on time and with eloquence, though their frequent flattering remarks about me belie the essential fact about all of this work: a team—a large team—of IHI colleagues and many others is behind every achievement I report or celebrate in these speeches. I continue to feel deeply grateful to the Institute for Healthcare Improvement, including its board, executives, staff, and faculty, for decades of support, mentoring, and encouragement of my efforts. Most of the ideas in these speeches came first from them, not me.

I offer special thanks to Maureen Bisognano, my successor as IHI CEO, and Tom Nolan, my mentor-in-chief, whose constant thoughtfulness has infused my work every step of the way.

And, last, thanks to my family—Ann, Ben, Beth, Dan, Jessica, Andrew, Becca, Joey, Nathaniel, Caleb, Bob, Sue, David, and Davy—who make it all worthwhile.

THE AUTHOR

DONALD M. BERWICK, MD, MPP, FRCP, is president emeritus and senior fellow at the Institute for Healthcare Improvement (IHI), an organization that Dr. Berwick cofounded and led as president and chief executive officer for eighteen years. He is one of the nation's leading authorities on health care quality and improvement. In July 2010, President Barack Obama appointed Dr. Berwick to the position of administrator of the Centers for Medicare & Medicaid Services (CMS), a position he held until December 2011. A pediatrician by background, Dr. Berwick has served as clinical professor of Pediatrics and Health Care Policy at the Harvard Medical School, professor of Health Policy and Management at the Harvard School of Public Health, and as a member of the staffs of Boston's Children's Hospital Medical Center, Massachusetts General Hospital, and the Brigham and Women's Hospital. He has also served as vice chair of the U.S. Preventive Services Task Force, the first "Independent Member" of the board of trustees of the American Hospital Association, and chair of the National Advisory Council of the Agency for Healthcare Research and Quality. An elected member of the Institute of Medicine (IOM), Dr. Berwick served two terms on the IOM's governing council and was a member of the IOM's Global Health Board. He served on President Bill Clinton's Advisory Commission on Consumer Protection and Quality in the Healthcare Industry.

He is a recipient of numerous awards, including the 1999 Joint Commission's Ernest Amory Codman Award, the 2002 American Hospital Association's Award of Honor, the 2006 John M. Eisenberg Patient Safety and Quality Award for Individual Achievement from the National Quality Forum and the Joint Commission on Accreditation of Healthcare Organizations, the 2007 William B. Graham Prize for Health Services Research, the 2007 Heinz Award for Public Policy from the Heinz Family Foundation, the 2012 Gustav O. Lienhard Award from the IOM, and the 2013 Nathan Davis Award from the American Medical Association. In 2005, he was appointed "Honorary Knight Commander of the British Empire" by Queen Elizabeth II, the highest honor awarded by the United Kingdom to non-British subjects, in recognition of his work with the British National Health Service.

Dr. Berwick is the author or coauthor of more than 160 scientific articles and four books. He also serves as lecturer in the Department of Health Care Policy at Harvard Medical School.

THE COMMENTARY AUTHORS

Chapter 1   My Right Knee

Gary S. Kaplan, MD, FACP, FACMPE, FACPE, has served as chairman and CEO of the Virginia Mason Health System in Seattle since 2000. Board certified in internal medicine, he is also a practicing internal medicine physician at Virginia Mason. During his tenure, Virginia Mason has received significant national and international praise for its efforts to transform health care, most notably as the leader in adapting the Toyota Production System for health care. Recognized as one of the most influential physician executives in health care, Dr. Kaplan has been honored nationally for his leadership. In 2009, he received the John M. Eisenberg Patient Safety and Quality Award for Individual Achievement from the National Quality Forum and the Joint Commission; and the Harry J. Harwick Lifetime Achievement Award from the Medical Group Management Association and the American College of Medical Practice Executives. Other accolades include being named on the *Modern Physician* and *Modern Healthcare* list of "50 Most Influential Physician Executives" in the United States eight times; *Modern Healthcare* 2012 list of the "100 Most Influential People in Healthcare"; and *Becker's Hospital Review* 2011 list of the "13 Most Influential Patient Safety Advocates in the United States" and one of the most important US "Health and Hospital Leaders to Know." Dr. Kaplan is a founding member of Health CEOs for Health Reform. He has held leadership positions with numerous organizations, including the National Patient Safety Foundation, the Medical Group Management Association, and the Washington Healthcare Forum. He is the chair of the Institute for Healthcare Improvement Board of Directors and the 2013–2014 chair of the Seattle Metropolitan Chamber of Commerce Board of Directors.

Chapter 2   Some Is Not a Number, Soon Is Not a Time

C. Joseph McCannon was senior advisor to the administrator at the Centers for Medicare & Medicaid Services (CMS), where he advised on agency policy, launched and led several large organizational initiatives to improve health care quality (including the Partnership for Patients), and was a member of the founding team at the Center for Medicare and Medicaid Innovation (CMMI). Previously, he served as vice president and faculty on dissemination and large-scale improvement at the Institute for Healthcare Improvement (IHI), where he also led organizational efforts to spread change in Africa, the United States, and several other regions. Mr. McCannon supported IHI's collaboration with the World Health Organization to design and amplify the "3 by 5" initiative, an effort to deliver antiretroviral drugs to three million people globally by the end of 2005. He also directed IHI's major US initiatives to improve patient safety—the 100,000 Lives Campaign and the 5 Million Lives Campaign—which involved more than four thousand hospitals and seventy field offices. He has advised or consulted to other national quality improvement efforts in the United States, England, Japan, Canada, and Denmark, and to initiatives outside of health care (for example, ending homelessness and corrections reform). His career began in the publishing industry with roles at *Fast Company*, the *Atlantic Monthly*, and *Outside* magazine. He is a graduate of Harvard University and was a Reuters and Merck Fellow at Stanford University in 2003–2004.

Chapter 3   Power

Dale Ann Micalizzi is a nationally known health care improvement advisor and trusted advocate for pediatric patient safety and transparency in medicine. Her eleven-year-old son, Justin, died following a "simple" incision and drainage of an infected ankle in 2001. She has worked tirelessly in search of answers about her son's death, giving rise to a quest to improve pediatric health care. Her efforts focus on compassion and support for grieving families, full disclosure of adverse medical events, and education and reform that will restore ethics and safety in medicine. She has presented as a faculty member for the Institute for Healthcare Improvement (IHI) beginning in 2005, and has acted as a consultant, speaker, board member, and improvement advisor for numerous health care organizations, medical schools, and patient/family support programs. Ms. Micalizzi is the founder and director of Justin's HOPE Project at the Task Force for Global Health, and she has partnered with IHI in providing yearly National Forum scholarships in Justin's memory to health caregivers who work with underserved pediatric populations internationally to improve safety and quality. She has channeled her grief, exacerbated by the absence of disclosure and apology, into programs that advance pediatric safety and educate a new generation about the importance of caring for families in the aftermath of tragic errors, learning from the event, and working with them to improve care together. She is coauthor of the chapter "The Heart of Health Care: Parents' Perspectives on Patient Safety" in *Pediatric Clinics of North America* and coauthor of an article in *Pediatric Anesthesia* titled "What Happens When Things Go Wrong?"

Chapter 4 Mont Sainte-Victoire

Jason Leitch, DDS, FDS, MPH, has worked for the Scottish government since 2007; he is currently the clinical director of the Quality Unit in the Health and Social Care Directorate. He is a member of the Health and Social Care Management Board and a member of the senior team responsible for implementation of the NHS Scotland Quality Strategy. He is also the medical director of the Tayside Centre for Organisational Effectiveness and an honorary professor at the University of Dundee. Professor Leitch was named the 2011 HFMA UK Clinician of the Year. He is a nonexecutive board member of AQuA in the North-East of England. He was a 2005–2006 Quality Improvement Fellow at the Institute for Healthcare Improvement (IHI), sponsored by the Health Foundation. He is also a trustee of the UK wing of the Indian Rural Evangelical Fellowship, which runs orphanages in southeast India. He has a doctorate from the University of Glasgow, an MPH from Harvard, and is a fellow of the Royal College of Surgeons of England, the Royal College of Physicians and Surgeons of Glasgow, and the Royal College of Surgeons of Edinburgh. He is also a fellow of the Higher Education Academy.

Chapter 5 A Message for Ramesh

Paul Farmer, MD, PhD, is Kolokotrones University Professor and chair of the Department of Global Health and Social Medicine at Harvard Medical School, chief of the Division of Global Health Equity at Brigham and Women's Hospital in Boston, and cofounder of Partners In Health. He also serves as UN special advisor to the secretary-general on Community Based Medicine and Lessons from Haiti. Dr. Farmer and his colleagues have pioneered novel, community-based treatment strategies that demonstrate the delivery of high-quality health care in resource-poor settings. He is a member of the Institute of Medicine of the National

Academy of Sciences and of the American Academy of Arts and Sciences. Dr. Farmer has written extensively on health, human rights, and the consequences of social inequality. His most recent book is *To Repair the World: Paul Farmer Speaks to the Next Generation*. Other titles include *Haiti After the Earthquake; Partner to the Poor: A Paul Farmer Reader; Pathologies of Power: Health, Human Rights, and the New War on the Poor; The Uses of Haiti; Infections and Inequalities: The Modern Plagues;* and *AIDS and Accusation: Haiti and the Geography of Blame*.

Chapter 6   Eating Soup with a Fork

Paul B. Batalden, MD, professor emeritus of Pediatrics, Community, and Family Medicine and the Dartmouth Institute for Health Policy and Clinical Practice at the Geisel School of Medicine at Dartmouth College, is also guest professor of Quality Improvement and Leadership at Jönköping University in Sweden. He teaches about the leadership of improvement of health care quality, safety, and value at Dartmouth, the Institute for Healthcare Improvement (IHI), and the Jönköping Academy for the Improvement of Health and Welfare in Sweden. He chairs the Improvement Science Development Group of the Health Foundation in London and the Leadership Preventive Medicine Residency Advisory Committee at Dartmouth. He is a member of the Board of Advisors, Armstrong Institute for Patient Safety and Quality, Johns Hopkins Medicine; the National Advisory Board, Active Aging Research Center, University of Wisconsin; External Advisory Council, Anderson Center, Cincinnati Children's Hospital and Medical Center; the Research and Education Board of Health Partners in St. Paul, Minnesota; and serves as senior fellow and governing board advisor for IHI. Previously he founded, created, or helped develop the IHI, the VA National Quality Scholars program, the IHI Health Professions Education Collaborative, the General Competencies of the ACGME, the Center for Leadership and Improvement at Dartmouth, the Dartmouth Hitchcock Leadership Preventive Medicine Residency, the annual health professional faculty development "summer camp," the SQUIRE publication guidelines for the improvement of health care, and the Improvement Science Fellowship Program of the Health Foundation in the UK and of the Vinnvård Improvement Science Fellowships in Sweden. He is a member of the Minnesota Academy of Medicine and the Institute of Medicine of the US National Academy of Sciences. He is currently interested in the multiple knowledge systems and disciplines that inform the improvement of health and health care.

Chapter 7 What "Patient-Centered" Should Mean: Confessions of an Extremist

Frederick S. Southwick, MD, received his BA from Yale College and his MD from Columbia College of Physicians and Surgeons. He received his clinical training at Boston City Hospital and the Massachusetts General Hospitals in Internal Medicine and Infectious Diseases, and served on the faculty at Harvard University and the University of Pennsylvania before serving as chief of Infectious Diseases at the University of Florida for nineteen years. Dr. Southwick has been an active NIH-funded biomedical investigator for more than thirty years, studying how bacteria interact with the human host. From 2010 to 2011, he was an Advanced Leadership Fellow at the Harvard Business School, where he studied leadership, teamwork, campaign strategies, and the principles of health care quality and safety. As part of his fellowship he completed a book entitled *Critically Ill: A 5-Point Plan to Cure Healthcare Delivery.* Most recently he was appointed quality projects manager for the senior vice president for Health Affairs at UF & Shands System.

Chapter 8 Tense

Jessica Berwick, MD, MPH, grew up in Newton, Massachusetts. She received her AB in government from Harvard College, an MD from Yale School of Medicine, and an MPH from Johns Hopkins Bloomberg School of Public Health. Throughout high school and college she spent time in Costa Rica, Ecuador, and Peru. She has worked at an HIV clinical trials site in Cape Town, South Africa, both during college and in the year preceding medical school. She has completed her training in Internal Medicine/Primary Care at Brigham and Women's Hospital. She is a hospitalist at Beth Israel Deaconness Medical Center, and plans to spend significant portions of her time working at the University of Zimbabwe College of Health Sciences in Harare, Zimbabwe. She is now living in Harare with her husband, Andrew, and her son, Nathaniel, dividing her time between Zimbabwe and the US.

Chapter 9 A Transatlantic Review of the NHS at Sixty

Lord Nigel Crisp is an independent crossbench member of the House of Lords in the United Kingdom, where he cochairs the All Party Parliamentary Group on Global Health. He was chief executive of the NHS in England—the largest health care organization in the world, with 1.4

million employees—and permanent secretary of the UK Department of Health between 2000 and 2006. Previously he was chief executive of the Oxford Radcliffe Hospital NHS Trust. Lord Crisp chairs Sightsavers, the Kings Partners Global Health Advisory Board, and the Zambian and Ugandan UK Health Alliances. He is a senior fellow of the Institute for Healthcare Improvement, and he is affiliated with the Harvard School of Public Health and the London School of Hygiene and Tropical Medicine. He has written extensively on health. His book *Turning the World Upside Down: The Search for Global Health in the 21st Century* takes further the ideas about partnership and mutual learning developed in his report for the prime minister, *Global Health Partnerships*.

Chapter 10   The Epitaph of Profession

Christine K. Cassel, MD, joined the National Quality Forum as president and CEO in July 2013. Previously, she served as president and CEO of the American Board of Internal Medicine (ABIM) and the ABIM Foundation. She is a leading expert in geriatric medicine, medical ethics, and quality of care. Dr. Cassel is a member of the President's Council of Advisors on Science and Technology (PCAST). She is the cochair and physician leader of PCAST working groups that have made recommendations to the president on issues relating to health information technology and ways to promote scientific innovation in drug development and evaluation. Dr. Cassel is a member of the Commonwealth Fund's Commission on a High Performance Health System and has served on the Institute of Medicine Committees that wrote the influential reports *To Err Is Human* and *Crossing the Quality Chasm*. She is an adjunct professor of medicine and senior fellow in the Department of Medical Ethics and Health Policy at the University of Pennsylvania School of Medicine, former dean of medicine at Oregon Health and Science University, chair of geriatrics at Mount Sinai School of Medicine in New York, and chief of General Internal Medicine at the University of Chicago. Dr. Cassel is a prolific scholar, having authored and edited fourteen books and more than two hundred published articles.

Chapter 11   Squirrel

Diana Chapman Walsh, PhD, president emerita, Wellesley College, serves on the governing boards of the Broad Institute of MIT and Harvard; the Kaiser Family Foundation; the Institute for Healthcare Improvement; the Massachusetts Institute of Technology; and the Mind and Life Institute; as well as on several national advisory boards. She was a director of the

State Street Corporation (1999 to 2007) and a trustee of Amherst College (1998 to 2010). A member of the American Academy of Arts and Sciences and Phi Beta Kappa, Dr. Walsh writes, speaks, and consults on higher education and leadership. Before assuming the Wellesley presidency, she was Norman Professor and Chair of Health and Social Behavior at the Harvard School of Public Health. Her tenure as twelfth president of Wellesley College (1993 to 2007) was marked by educational innovation, including a revision of the curriculum and expanded programs in global education, the humanities, internships and service learning, interdisciplinary teaching and learning, and religious and spiritual life. President Walsh evolved a distinctive style of reflective leadership rooted in a network of resilient partnerships and anchored in the belief that trustworthy leadership starts from within.

Chapter 12   You Decide

Beverley H. Johnson is president and CEO of the Institute for Patient- and Family-Centered Care in Bethesda, Maryland. She has provided technical assistance to more than 250 hospitals, health systems, primary care practices, and federal, state, and provincial agencies. She has authored and coauthored many publications on patient- and family-centered practice. She recently served as project director for a multiyear initiative to develop resource materials for senior leaders in hospital, ambulatory, and long-term care settings on how to partner with patients, residents, and families to enhance the quality, safety, and the experience of care. Ms. Johnson serves on the selection committee for the American Hospital Association-McKesson Quest for Quality Prize and is a member of the Patient-Centered Primary Care Collaborative Board of Directors. She is also a member of Premier's QUEST/PACT Advisory Panel and the American College of Physicians' Advisory Board for Patient Partnership in Healthcare. She was presented with the Humanitarian Award by Pediatric Nursing in 1990, and the Lloyd Bentsen Award in 1992. In 2007, she was honored with The Changemaker Award by the Board for the Center for Health Care Design and the Gravens Award for leadership in promoting optimal environments and developmental care for high-risk infants and their families. She is also a recipient of the Dorland Health 2011 People Award.

Chapter 13   The Moral Test

Tom Daschle is a senior policy advisor to the law firm DLA Piper, where he provides strategic advice on public policy issues such as climate change, energy, health care, trade, financial services, and telecommunications. In 2007, he joined with former Senate Majority Leaders George Mitchell, Bob Dole, and Howard Baker to form the Bipartisan Policy Center, an organization dedicated to finding common ground on some of the most pressing public policy issues of our time. Senator Daschle is also the vice chair of the National Democratic Institute and a board member of the Center for American Progress. He is the author of the books *Like No Other Time: The 107th Congress and the Two Years That Changed America Forever*; *Critical: What We Can Do About the Health-Care Crisis*; *Getting It Done: How Obama and Congress Finally Broke the Stalemate to Make Way for Health Reform*; and *The US Senate: Fundamentals of American Government*. He is a graduate of South Dakota State University.

Chapter 14   New Health System—New Professionalism

James Reason, PhD, graduated from the University of Manchester in 1962 and received his PhD from the University of Leicester in 1967. He was professor of psychology at Manchester from 1976 to 2001, and is now emeritus professor. His main research area has been the human contribution both to accidents in complex technological systems and to recovering these systems when they slide towards disaster. He is best known for his "Swiss Cheese" model of accident causation. Dr. Reason has consulted in many hazardous domains, but recently he has focused on patient safety. He has authored or coauthored more than a dozen books and several journal articles. His most recent book is *A Life in Error*. He is a fellow of the British Academy, the Royal Aeronautical Society, the Royal College of General Practitioners, and the British Psychological Society. He is married with two daughters and three grandchildren.

Chapter 15   To Isaiah

Mark D. Smith, MD, MBA, has been president and chief executive officer of the California HealthCare Foundation (CHCF) since its founding in 1996 until 2013. CHCF is an independent philanthropy headquartered in Oakland, California, that is dedicated to improving the health of the people of California, with special concern for the underserved. A board-certified internist, Dr. Smith is a member of the clinical faculty at the University of California, San Francisco, and an attending physician at the Positive Health Program for AIDS Care at San Francisco General

Hospital. He is a member of the Institute of Medicine, National Academy of Sciences, and chaired the Committee on the Learning Healthcare System in America. He has served on the Performance Measurement Committee of the National Committee for Quality Assurance, the National Business Group on Health Board of Directors, and the editorial board of the *Annals of Internal Medicine*. He is author of *On Practical Progress*. Dr. Smith received a bachelor's degree from Harvard College, an MD from the University of North Carolina at Chapel Hill, and an MBA from the Wharton School at the University of Pennsylvania.

Chapter 16   And We Said, "No"

Patricia A. Gabow, MD, was CEO of Denver Health from 1992 until her retirement in 2012, transforming it from a department of city government to a successful, independent governmental entity. She is a member of the Medicaid and CHIP Access and Payment Commission (MACPAC), the Robert Wood Johnson Foundation Board, the Institute of Medicine Roundtable on Value and Science Driven Health Care, and the National Governors Association Health Advisory Board. She is a professor of medicine at the University of Colorado School of Medicine and has authored more than 150 articles and book chapters. She received her MD degree from the University of Pennsylvania School of Medicine. She trained in Internal Medicine and Nephrology at the Hospital of the University of Pennsylvania, Harbor General Hospital, and San Francisco General Hospital. Dr. Gabow has received the AMA Nathan Davis Award for Outstanding Public Servant, the Ohtli Award from the Mexican government, the National Healthcare Leadership Award, the David E. Rogers Award from AAMC, the Health Quality Leader Award from NCQA, and was elected to the Association for Manufacturing Excellence Hall of Fame for her work on Toyota Production Systems in health care.

INTRODUCTION

IN HIS PREFACE, Don talks about the role serendipity played in connecting him with so many influential and inspiring people—both in his life and his career. I have a slightly different take. I agree that serendipity and circumstance have been pivotal, but his accomplishments and impact are by no means accidental. For me, it's not so much *who* Don has interacted with as it is *how* he engages them. It's how he engages patients, like Isaiah, and like all those he has met in his "second" career as a health care leader. It's how he engages other leaders—from health care systems and from governments all over the world. And, perhaps most important, it's how he engages caregivers—the people at the point of care, whose devotion and commitment to the patients they care for forms the heart of health care and inspires us all to improve.

In all these interactions, from those with government leaders to those with front-line staff, the two words that best characterize the nature of Don's engagement are, for me, *humanity* and *humility*. Roles aren't important to Don . . . people are. He approaches everyone as a person first, a whole person. His curiosity is about the humanity in each of us and how that drives us all to be better caregivers, better leaders, and better colleagues. He knows how to get the best from each of us and how to honor and use the assets we all have. And he does this always with a genuine humility—the kind of humility he displays in his Preface, and the humility that runs throughout all of these collected speeches. Don always wants to be a member of a team, of a movement. He knows that *collective* action is the key to system transformation, and that everyone has a crucial role to play.

I first met Don in 1987, when I was a new CEO at a Massachusetts hospital, and he invited me to join the National Demonstration Project on Quality Improvement in Health Care—the NDP, for short. I was young, and green, and a bit daunted by the opportunity to join improvement's pioneers—Blan Godfrey, Paul Batalden, and Don—to learn how we might best improve health care by taking lessons from outside the industry. My own mentors at the time were from Florida Power & Light, a utility company in Miami. They taught me how to innovate and improve, and they set me on the path that, serendipitously, crossed Don's and changed my life.

In those early days, Don coached, inspired, and taught. But he also always listened, learned, and honored. Whether he's tracking down Isaiah to follow up on his blood work or launching a national campaign to save lives, Don begins by first understanding the strengths and capabilities of all, and then capturing them with his own enthusiasm and passion.

The National Demonstration Project brought twenty-one hospitals together with twenty industry leaders outside of health care to learn together about quality, safety, customer satisfaction, and cost. The leaders engaged in the project saw real improvements. And the lessons they learned and momentum they generated formed the foundation for what became the Institute for Healthcare Improvement—a foundation still solid some twenty-five years later.

I will say this: Don does have his limits. He hits the wall when he sees injustice, indifference, or complacency. In these assembled speeches, as with the earlier collection, *Escape Fire* (2004), you can feel his impatience with the health care system as it is. He sees that the medical systems we have don't reliably contribute to health, that care sometimes harms, and that it all costs far too much. You can feel his frustration when the patient's voice isn't heard or when illogical rules—like visiting hours—keep loved ones apart. Through these speeches, Don inspires us to make our systems better, make them more effective, and make them more humane.

Don's is the needed voice for reforming health care. The Triple Aim concept, which he codesigned with John Whittington and Tom Nolan, is pushing us to improve the health of populations, to improve the experience of care, and to reduce per capita costs. He defines this agenda as our "moral test," and pulls us all to this vision, over the rough roads of payment disincentives, regulatory complexity, professional silos, and fragmented systems. He does this in two important ways. Above all, Don gives us the heart and courage we need if we are going to change. He puts the voices and faces of patients before us and dares us to walk away from their need. He defines compassion for each other, and the joys we can find in working together. He tells us about patients like Isaiah to open our eyes to the meaning of life, health, and caring. He puts the hard choice to us: to change, or not to change.

And he also gives us science, systems theory, tools, and mechanisms to support us once we set our ambitious aims. The stories in these speeches describe data, scientific approaches, and new models to innovate and improve. He defines the ways policy and regulation can support change. He shows us the way to see systems and pathways across complex organizational barriers. He teaches how to use science and data and evaluation for improvement, not for judgment.

I've been to every National Forum since the first one in 1989. And though there are thousands of others in the room, I always look forward to Don's talk as his hour with me. I know I'm not alone in feeling this. He connects with our individuality, with our uniqueness. But then the lights come up, and the audience stands (they always stand), and I'm reminded that I'm part of something big, something greater than myself. Don reminds us all, those in the room, and the thousands more watching from all corners of the globe, that we are one big team, with one common mission: we have to rescue health care by improving it.

I've had the honor to watch Don write and refine these speeches, the privilege to be a sounding board and reviewer, and the joyful opportunity to hear most of them delivered in person. And as wonderful as these speeches are on their own, the commentaries that accompany them are just as extraordinary. It's telling that among this group of luminaries who contributed their thoughts and impressions, not one of them hesitated when invited to write a commentary. I'm sure they felt just as flattered and humbled as I did when asked to write this introduction. Don has that effect on people.

With this book, Don will once again inspire and teach the world. He'll help you renew your promise to Isaiah, see your Baby Gray, find your Ramesh Kumar, answer the question, "What do you really, really want?," and help us all find the courage and wisdom to make health care better, safer, and more efficient. You'll never sit by a patient's bedside without feeling what empathic caring can be like. You'll never feel alone in pointing out a system fault and suggesting a possible solution. You might even start to understand what it feels like to root for the Boston Red Sox. Enjoy!

MAUREEN BISOGNANO
President and CEO
Institute for Healthcare Improvement

PROMISING CARE

Chapter 1

MY RIGHT KNEE

COMMENTARY

Gary S. Kaplan, MD

AT THE INSTITUTE for Healthcare Improvement (IHI) National Forum in 2003, then-President and CEO Don Berwick, MD, gave a keynote speech titled "My Right Knee." I always look forward to hearing Don speak, but I wasn't quite prepared to hear a speech that would provide a defining moment in my own leadership journey and quest for quality. His keynote was a mandate for transformational change in health care.

I have known Don for decades and, in addition to my service as chairman and CEO of Virginia Mason Health System in Seattle, I am proud to serve as the current chair of the IHI Board of Directors. In 2003, the team at Virginia Mason was in the very early stages of adopting the Toyota Production System as our management method. We were intrigued by this system because it is sharply focused on achieving perfect quality. Although zero defects is an admirable goal, many said it was impossible. After all, Virginia Mason is in the business of providing health care, not manufacturing cars.

It was Don's description of his own experience in search of high-quality, patient-focused care, and the disappointments and successes he experienced along the way, that gave me courage to stay the course in pursuit of the perfect patient experience.

Don's vision was that radical transformation was not possible until "we look at the people we want to help, and see ourselves; when we realize that their needs, out there, are our needs, in here." His insistence that we view health care through the eyes of our patients prompted my own thoughts of my parents, my wife, my children, and my future grandchildren. This was confirmation that zero defects is the only acceptable goal in health care.

A baseball fan (a gross understatement), Don tied the likelihood of whole-system transformation in health care to the chances of the Boston Red Sox winning the World Series. So, what has happened in the decade since Don gave that pivotal speech? The Red Sox won the World Series—twice—in 2004 and again in 2007. What seemed like an unlikely accomplishment on the baseball field was a harbinger of things to come in health care.

IHI continued to drive improvement in health care quality and safety with its groundbreaking 100,000 Lives and 5 Million Lives Campaigns, motivating hospitals across America to significantly reduce morbidity, mortality, and errors in health care by adopting practices focused on patient safety.

For organizations faced with interpreting the Institute of Medicine's (IOM) landmark report, *Crossing the Quality Chasm: A New Health System for the 21st Century*, IHI created the clarity we needed in health care to engage in this work by reframing the IOM aims for improvement—care that is safe, effective, patient-centered, timely, efficient, and equitable—as "no needless pain, no needless death, and no needless waste." This mantra became the rallying cry for whole-system change in health care.

In addition to its work in the United States, IHI continued to expand its international reach. The Surviving Sepsis Campaign, in partnership with IHI, developed international guidelines for the management of severe sepsis and septic shock. Further, IHI's work with the World Health Organization (WHO) includes the promotion and spread of WHO's important surgical safety programs.

Throughout the country, we are now implementing the Patient Protection and Affordable Care Act, and with IHI providing successful models, we are seeing health care–associated infections and hospital readmissions decrease. At the same time we are providing more preventive care with better coordination through increased use of electronic medical records.

A decade after Don's speech, organizations like Virginia Mason continue to experience what it means to be a learning organization. We do this by employing a management method, the Virginia Mason Production System, that insists on patient-focused alignment throughout our health system. This pursuit of the perfect patient experience requires transparency and a focus on respect for our patients as team members. As Don revealed, the only way we can achieve this is by walking in our patients' shoes.

"My Right Knee" was a personal turning point for me, and it raised the bar for the health care industry. Ten years later, are we where we need to be, ensuring no needless pain, no needless death, and no needless waste? Honestly, no. Yet the Red Sox did win the World Series, proving there is a cure for the curse of the Bambino. Similarly, I believe there is a cure for what ails health care.

MY RIGHT KNEE

PLENARY ADDRESS
INSTITUTE FOR HEALTHCARE IMPROVEMENT
15TH ANNUAL NATIONAL FORUM ON QUALITY
IMPROVEMENT IN HEALTH CARE
NEW ORLEANS, LOUISIANA, DECEMBER 4, 2003

A DARK CLOUD hangs over IHI's home base, Boston, this year. It's the cloud of the Boston Red Sox. This is very painful for us, and especially for Maureen Bisognano, my closest colleague and IHI's brilliant executive vice president and COO. Maureen is as avid a Red Sox fan as she is a golfer. That's saying a lot, if you know about Maureen and golf. Just this fall, she phoned me after a weekend round of golf to say that it had been terrible. She was on the third tee when her golfing partner, Fred, dropped dead of a heart attack.

I said, "Maureen, that must have been so hard for you."

"You have no idea how hard it was," she said. "It took forever . . . hit the ball, drag Fred, hit the ball, drag Fred. . . ."

So, Maureen was a mess when, again, the Red Sox, her beloved team, got knocked out of the semi-final round—the American League Championship Series—by our archrivals, the New York Yankees, Satan's team. We came so close.

If you're not from the United States, let me explain. The Boston Red Sox suffer from a problem we call the "curse of the Bambino." "The Bambino" is Babe Ruth—it's his nickname—who was probably the great-

---

Note: This speech was published subsequently, by *Annals of Internal Medicine*, as "My Right Knee." (Berwick DM. My right knee. *Ann Int Med*, 2005 Jan;142(2): 121–125. http://annals.org/article.aspx?articleid=718104)

est baseball player of all time. Babe Ruth started his professional career with the Red Sox, but in 1920, in search of filthy lucre, the owner of the Red Sox sold the Babe to the New York Yankees, Satan's team. With Babe Ruth on board, the Red Sox won the baseball championship, which we Americans humbly call the World Series, in 1918, but they haven't ever won it since. Meanwhile the Yankees have won the World Series twenty-six times. Bostonians know that the gods, themselves, have engineered this century of failure for the Red Sox—always a bridesmaid, never a bride—because of that treacherous trade; so they call it the "curse of the Bambino."

The Red Sox have fixed this problem lots of times, not by winning the World Series, but by firing people. In a famous instant in the 1986 World Series—Red Sox versus the New York Mets, Satan's other team—oh, it is seared in my sons' memories, and don't even *think* of mentioning it to Maureen—our first baseman, Bill Buckner, muffed an easy ground ball, and the Mets went on to beat us. Buckner was gone the next year. This year, in the seventh and final game of the American League playoffs, the Red Sox manager, Grady Little, left our worn-out star pitcher in one inning too long, and that let the Yankees come back from way behind to beat us. Grady Little is now the *former* manager of the Red Sox. That'll fix it!

This all has led to a common bet in Boston: people bet on which will happen first—"X" or the Red Sox winning the World Series. Graduate students' supervisors ask them if they'll finish their PhD theses before the Red Sox win the World Series. Their mothers ask them if they'll get married before the Red Sox win the World Series. I ask my kids if they'll please clean their rooms before the Red Sox win the World Series. I intend to empty my email inbox before the Red Sox win the World Series.

So, in that spirit, I ask you here: Which will happen first, the health care we ought to have, or the Red Sox winning the World Series? Being a health care improvement fan and a Boston Red Sox fan do have something in common: playoffs, but no Series. Until recently, I would have bet on the Red Sox.

But, now, I'm not so sure. It's been a good year for the quality movement . . . a very good year. I think a real turning point was actually almost exactly one year ago, when Sister Mary Jean Ryan and her colleagues at SSM Health Care earned and won the Malcolm Baldrige National Quality Award. They met world-class quality standards with the best assessment criteria we have on the same playing field as other industries! Now we have the news that two more places have followed in SSM's steps: Baptist Hospital in Pensacola and St. Luke's in Kansas City just won the Baldrige, too.

The IHI had a good year. We launched our new IMPACT network—I call it "The Association for Change." A new project supported by the Robert Wood Johnson Foundation, called Transforming Care at the Bedside, is part of IHI's growing focus on helping the nursing profession—something we just have to tackle as a top priority in American health care.

Our Pursuing Perfection project, also funded by the Robert Wood Johnson Foundation, has begun to show major gains in all thirteen sites—seven US and six European. Maybe best of all, I am now clearly seeing a small but increasing number of American health care organizations finally aiming for whole system change—what we've been waiting for: improvement as the core strategy. For example, Randy Linton and his colleagues at Luther Midelfort; John Toussaint and Scott Decker at ThedaCare; George Kerwin and Pete Knox at Bellin Health System in Wisconsin; Gary Kaplan at Virginia Mason in Seattle; Sister Mary Jean and SSM throughout the country; Leo Brideau at Columbia St. Mary's in Milwaukee; Mayo Clinic at all of its sites; Bill Corley at Community Hospitals in Indianapolis; and Doug Eby and his colleagues at the Southcentral Foundation and the Alaska Native Medical Center in Anchorage; to name only a few.

And, the improvement movement is now absolutely global. Sweden, Norway, the UK, the Netherlands, Australia, and New Zealand are only some of the bright spots. The UK improvements are soaring with the help of such leaders and IHI friends as Sir Liam Donaldson, Sir Brian Jarman, David Fillingham, and Helen Bevan. John Oldham, longtime friend, associate, and senior faculty member of the IHI, was knighted this year—he is now Sir John Oldham, but he lets me call him, simply, "Sir"—because of what he's done to improve the UK's primary care services. The IHI is now working with the World Health Organization to figure out how to expand our efforts into the fight against AIDS.

Federal agencies are also doing tons. Take a look at Medicare, with some bold, new programs to reward exceptional quality of care, led by Steve Jencks, Sean Tunis, Barbara Paul, and Michael McMullin; the Bureau of Primary Health Care in HRSA, showing massive improvements in access and chronic disease care in community health centers under the leadership of Sam Shekar; and the Veterans Health Administration, setting the pace in patient safety.

Trying to keep up with this pace of change, IHI's management team and staff have been working this year on a big redesign of the IHI itself. We've decided that we're going to focus all of our energies—that we'll judge ourselves—on what we are actually achieving on the Institute of Medicine's [IOM] six aims for improvement: safety, effectiveness, patient-centeredness, timeliness, efficiency, and equity. We are going to make IHI more results oriented than ever before.

We have rephrased the IOM's aims a little. Here are the results we want to get, and we want to get them with you:

- No needless death
- No needless pain
- No helplessness
- No unwanted waiting
- No waste

And we want those results for all—for everyone; that's the sixth IOM dimension: equity. That's what IHI exists to accomplish. That's how we'll measure our progress and yours. This clarifies our priorities. We will work on what helps get there, and we will turn down chances to work on things that don't.

So, with all of this, I'm bullish on improvement. It's a tight playoff series, but quality is pulling ahead by a game or two. Maybe, just maybe, the curse of the chasm—the health care quality chasm—will fall before the curse of the Bambino does. The trick now, just like for the Red Sox, is to put it all together.

This year, the stakes on that race—the race to put it all together—are up for me. Pretty soon, for me, what's been a spectator sport is going to be a participant one. I'll explain in a minute.

But, first, let me tell you a story.

This is my favorite saying; it comes from Mahatma Gandhi: "You must be the change you wish to see in the world." My colleague, Manoj Jain, from Tennessee, told me the following story about Gandhi that makes the point clearer.

The story is about a ten-year-old boy, Anil. Anil had become obese and was showing early signs of diabetes. His mother was at the end of her rope, and so she took Anil to Gandhi and asked the great man to tell Anil to stop eating sweets—no cakes, no pies, no candy. It could save his life. But, Gandhi refused. He said, "I can't do that. You'll have to come back in fifteen days."

"But, why not, Gandhiji?" the confused mother asked.

Gandhi said again, "Come back in fifteen days." And so she left with Anil, disappointed.

She returned as Gandhi asked, with Anil, after fifteen days, and then Gandhi sat with the boy and talked quietly.

"But, why couldn't you have done that fifteen days ago, Gandhiji?" the mother asked.

"Because fifteen days ago," Gandhi said, "I, too, was eating cakes, and pies, and candy. Now I have stopped, and I can tell Anil that I won't start eating them again until he can."

Isn't that an interesting idea? Helping by joining. A little scary, though.

The problem we need to solve is this: despite the good news, no one seems yet to have put it all together for the total quality of care—like the Red Sox, real, transformation change is still a bridesmaid, not a bride. It must be very hard to get there—to total quality. It must take some different level of energy, insight, and courage than we've mustered so far. But, I think I have an idea about how we can do it, and that's what I want to talk with you about—where the courage is.

I propose this: if we are going to care enough to do it all—to win the series—really, really different care—we're going to have to change the way we see our patients' lives, not as movies, out there, but as mirrors, in here. We'll change when we look at the people we want to help, and see ourselves; when we realize that their needs, out there, are our needs, in here. When we realize that the white coat and the dark suit are disguises. I am toying with the idea that our next, big step is not just to serve people but to join them. Gandhi joined Anil.

Take a risk with me. Ask yourself what health care you or a loved one might need between now and when the Red Sox win the World Series. Don't do it hypothetically—ask it for real. Some of you know, but most of you don't. But you can guess. What need will you have? How might you suffer? What will you need?

You have the next two days here at IHI's National Forum to design exactly the care you're going to want. That's going to take courage—to drop your guard, to be a patient, to understand what you need. But, I hereby declare that, for the next two days, you have a right to demand the help you want, when you want it, the way you want it. And, I'm going to go first.

This is my right knee. It is on your left . . . my right (which already worries me).

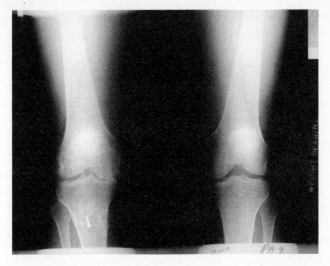

**Radiograph of the Author's Knees, Showing
"Bone-on-Bone" Osteoarthritis of the Right Knee**

I was born with two knees. Now, I have maybe 1.7 knees. It all started
when I was in medical school. Playing soccer one day, my right kneecap
"subluxed" or dislocated for an instant toward the outside of my knee,
and then flipped back into place. That hurt. When it happened again, I
went to see a surgeon. He said that my knee mechanics weren't lined up
right, and that I needed an operation. I was a nerd in medical school—
hard to believe, I know—and so I had read up on myself in advance, and
asked him if he thought an operation that I think was called the McRae
procedure would be a good one. He said, "Fine," and so I had the operation a few weeks later.

Oh, my goodness! I remember the pain when I woke up. It was so bad
that, for a minute, I couldn't even feel it. It was like a big truck so close
to my face that I couldn't tell at first that it was a truck. Then, the truck
hit me—for about two days—pain absolutely nothing like the soreness
of a subluxing kneecap. Not even on the same continent of pain.

But, I trusted medicine, and so I went through it with what I'd call
"writhing optimism"—since at least my problem was now over. It sort
of was over. My kneecap never again subluxed to the outside of my knee;
a few weeks later, it subluxed to the inside of my knee.

So I went back to see the surgeon. He was apologetic; he said that he
had apparently overcorrected the problem. I agreed politely. I asked him

if he had ever seen that before. He said, no, actually, because that was the first time he had ever done that particular operation, something he hadn't mentioned to me before it all started. "Maybe I should have told you," he said. I agreed politely. Within a few years, by the way, when it was finally subjected to a long-term follow-up study, the McRae procedure for my kind of problem was discredited—its complication rate was something like 30 percent.

So, I went to another surgeon at a different hospital—a community hospital near where I grew up. The surgeon there was happy to help. He suggested a simple repair job, which went pretty well, except for a couple of days of shaking chills and temperature of 104 degrees postoperatively. At least my knee never subluxed again.

That was that for twenty years. At age forty-five, I was playing basketball with my kids when my knee—the same one—suddenly gave way and exploded in pain. A bunch of tests followed—X-rays, MRIs, CAT scans—but no diagnosis. Everything looked okay, the local orthopedist said, except that I couldn't walk.

I was a little bit frustrated, so I went to a sports medicine clinic in another city, where I had seen some terrific improvement work, and saw a specialist I admired. He agreed that the tests didn't show anything, but his clinical impression was that I had torn a cartilage and needed arthroscopic surgery. He did it—no pain this time, by the way—found the cartilage tear, and trimmed it.

That did the trick, so well in fact that I increased my jogging and five years later, in 1998, I ran the Boston Marathon for the first and last time. My friend says that, given my knee history, this shows that I have the courage of a lion and the brain of a gerbil. I agreed politely. It was my only marathon because, during it, I blew out my cartilage again, and ended up on the arthroscopy table for the second time—my fourth knee operation—losing most of the damaged cartilage.

Now, eight years later, my knee has pretty much had it. The cushioning cartilage on the inside half of the joint is completely gone. I have, in the poetry of the orthopedic surgical literature, "bone on bone," which is a bad thing in a joint, where it's supposed to be "cartilage on cartilage."

Bone wears down; cartilage doesn't. I don't know when, but sometime, pretty soon, I am going to need a total knee replacement—maybe even to walk, but certainly to do the things I love to do outside, like hike and cross-country ski and climb. Frankly, I don't think I can hold out until the Red Sox win the World Series.

But here—long way around—is my problem: I'm scared. Actually, I'm terrified. That's not a rhetorical statement; it's a fact. I know that my future function is going to depend on taking advantage of this amazing technology—total knee replacement—but I also know much too much, much more than I want to know, about what could go wrong.

I told you that the IHI is trying to focus on five goals for health care change in the world: no needless death, no needless pain, no helplessness, no unwanted waiting, and no waste. At a system level, these are a vision. At a personal level, that is, for my knee and me, they're more than a vision—they're a need.

So, I had a meeting with my knee, and we decided to issue an RFP—a Request for Proposals—like a foundation does when it wants some research done, or like a company does when it wants a contract. My knee and I want to get some bids. We'll set the specs, and then anyone who wants to can bid to get the job.

My specs are the same as the IHI's vision: the "No needless" list. But, since it's my own knee—or 0.7 of a knee—I'll need to adapt the RFP with a little more detail.

Specification Number One Is "No Needless Deaths"

My RFP says it this way: "Don't kill me." At first, I wrote, "*Please* don't kill me," but then I decided to be a little more assertive. What do you think?

Prospective applicants: I'm warning you that I don't take this deliverable for granted. When I give you the contract on my knee, it will, absolutely, be a little bit like what the mafia also calls "a contract"—on my life. You become 007, licensed to kill . . . me. You see, the minute I slip under your anesthetic and your knife, I will, without any doubt, be taking the greatest risk to my life, statistically, that I have ever taken—greater by at least one order of magnitude, maybe two. I have climbed Mt. Rainier, crevassed and with vicious weather, five times. On those five climbs combined, I was running a risk of dying, if you use historical figures, one-fiftieth as great as I will take in your operating room. Each airplane flight I take will be five thousand times less lethal than my flight through your operating room.

Here is how you can kill me. Actually, there are too many ways for me to list them all, but here are some of the ways you can kill me. You can give me an infection during my surgery. You can mix up a blood transfusion if I need blood. You can fail to prevent my pulmonary embolism. If I need a respirator for a while when I wake up, you can give me pneumonia. You can forget that I am allergic to hazelnuts and maybe to codeine. You can misplace a decimal point in the order for morphine.

You can place the endotracheal tube by mistake in my esophagus, and not realize it until it's too late.

Everything on that list, by the way, happens and can be prevented—not down to zero, but awfully close to zero—I'll call it "Mt. Rainier" close to zero. I'm not asking you to make me as safe in your care as I am in my home, just please make me as safe in your care as when I cross the crevassed glaciers of Mt. Rainier.

I can give you some hints about how to do this. You can bring my surgical site infection rate as low as Baptist DeSoto Hospital or LDS Hospital has. You can prevent deep vein thrombosis and ventilator-acquired pneumonia as completely as Dominican Santa Cruz and Baptist DeSoto. You can be as attentive to medication errors as OSF, and you can use the VA's approach to preventing esophageal intubations—which in America average 8 percent of all non-critical-care intubations.

Without my RFP, I'd be entering the lottery of safety that we now have in this country. Four years ago, I sat in a room with about thirty hospital CEOs as they were shown their complication rates for, of all things, total knee and total hip replacement in their own hospitals. The rate of complications ranged from 3 percent in the lowest hospital to 21 percent in the highest. Now—forget about the 21 percent—even 3 percent doesn't feel all that good to me, frankly. If I told you that you were about to do something that stood one chance in thirty of hurting you really badly, would you do it? But, beyond that, I have to tell you that, as far as I know, no member of the public had access to that information at the time, or since. In my RFP, I am going to ask you to please tell me how you are doing, and, if you don't tell me, then I have to assume that either you don't know or that maybe you have something to hide. I don't mean to be strident or rude, but I really don't think you have a right not to tell me your results and then expect me to give you my knee to work on.

Actually, I've been there, done that. That's sort of what that very nice first orthopedic surgeon tried with me. He did an operation he had never done before, and he couldn't possibly have known the chances it would help or hurt me, beyond a wild guess. If that's what was going on, he should have told me. He was very nice, but he should have told me.

You might kill me. I want you to promise me that you know that. And, I want you to promise me that you've done everything you possibly can to reduce that risk to its theoretical minimum. None of my children are married yet; I haven't met my first grandchild yet; my wife and I want to take a trip to Nunavit someday; and I want to hike in the Himalayas. Now that I think of it, I want to watch my son's faces—Ben's and Dan's faces—when the Red Sox win the World Series, and I want to go to the party Maureen is going to throw that night. And, if you take that stuff away from me by killing me, I will be very, very upset with you.

Specification Number Two in the RFP Is "No Needless Pain"

Now, I have to explain this one, too, in my own terms. It means, "Assuming you don't kill me, don't hurt me either."

I know that's a little unrealistic, because, after all, surgery is itself a form of hurting. I accept that. I'm not asking for perfect; I am asking for the least possible harm. I want you to know what's the least possible harm, anywhere, and get it for me. Specification Number Two has three subparts, actually, which I call 2A, 2B, and 2C.

Specification 2A is "Don't do stuff to me that won't help me." I have a track record on this one. As it happens, I don't think that I ever needed surgery on my knee in the first place. I certainly didn't need the extensive, painful, since-discredited procedure that this guy tried on me for his first time. The subluxation problem I had was pretty minimal, and now I think that a brace and some exercises would have been enough. I think I fell into the very trap that Jack Wennberg has been trying to point out to us for over two decades: that, in health care, supply drives demand, without regard to the quality of outcomes of care. Wennberg's work, now beautifully extended by his protégé Elliott Fisher, shows that, at American levels of supply of specialty services, we can find no evidence at all that increasing supply produces better outcomes for patients at a population level—just more use and more cost.

Dr. Fisher's brilliant recent *Annals of Internal Medicine* paper shows that if you divide American hospital service areas into quintiles according to the intensity of their services—from the lowest quintile, the lowest 20 percent, to the highest one, the highest 20 percent—and then you study the quality of care in each area several different ways, such as finding out if people reliably get the care that can help them, here's what you find: quality doesn't change at all with quintile. More intensity doesn't get you any more quality of care until you reach the top quintile—the most cost, the most intensity—and there, for some important measures, quality *decreases*. More is not better. At the top level, outcomes are worse. This is a frightening finding, with imponderably large implications for American health care. In fact, nobody powerful in American health care seems to want to touch this one yet with a ten-foot pole.

It is scary for me to think about it, but if Wennberg and Fisher are right, the reason my first knee operation was done in the first place may well have been not because my knee *problem* was there, but because the knee *surgeon* was there. In fact, the same surgeon examined my other knee at the same time, said it was "tracking poorly" and probably should be operated on sometime to prevent subluxing. Happily, we never got around to that, and my left knee is just fine. That makes me also believe that the first surgery probably had something to do with causing the later cartilage problems. Maybe not.

Do I believe for a minute that that kind surgeon secretly rubbed his hands together greedily and cackled, "Hee, hee, hee—another knee I can make money on—little does this poor medical student nerd know . . ."? Not on your life. Absolutely not. I'd bet my life—actually, I did bet my life, didn't I?—that that surgeon believed that he was going to do me good. I am sure of that.

But, the fact remains: now I know that I had useless surgery for a nonsurgical problem. My surgeon and I didn't know that then. I have a screw in my knee for no good reason at all. My knee got screwed unnecessarily.

Specification 2B is "Don't do that again." I don't want a single drug, test, visit, stitch, or exercise regime that doesn't help me. You hurt me when you do that. I want you to promise that you don't do unproven, unnecessary things to me. Act on evidence, not just on hope.

Specification 2C is "Reduce the suffering I have from my bad knee." It's the obverse of Spec 2A. Reduce the burden of disease. That's why I am coming to you in the first place. It's Job 2, just behind safety. This is a balance, I know; I can handle that. Maybe you could offer me a higher chance of great function with a new prosthesis that is a little less tested than the old standby, but slightly more promising. I can understand that sometimes risks and results are a trade-off. What I want you to do is to involve me in that trade-off decision. I can help you make it, but only if you let me help you make it.

Now, once we've decided on what to do, do it right, please. Don't add to my pain by a complication, and please do choose your approach to anesthesia, prosthetic implant, postoperative recovery, and so on based on science. Since my right knee is on your left, and vice versa, I want to make sure that you don't get your signals crossed on that while I am asleep. I will give you credit if your response to my RFP tells me how you make sure to execute this clinical plan absolutely reliably. I won't give you a lot of credit for telling me that you value autonomy for your nurses and doctors if that means you don't use scientific evidence reliably. I take off points for wide variations in your clinical protocols from doctor to doctor.

Here's a question I'd like you to answer. Suppose the doctor who was meant to operate on me Tuesday morning got the flu on Monday, and so a different doctor had to do the operation. Would you guarantee to me that the same high level of quality of care—the exact same, evidence-based care—will happen anyway? When I got on the airplane to fly here from Boston on Monday, I didn't need to know the name of the pilot to have confidence in the trip. I want it to be the same on your operating table.

This has a lot to do with your culture. Is it open and fair, and does it value input from anyone in the know? Let me tell you a little detour story. A year or two ago, trying to plan ahead for a better knee, I went to see a surgeon who several friends told me was a young up-and-comer—let's call him "Dr. Upandcomer"—who told me he could help by doing a semi-experimental procedure involving removing a wedge of bone from my tibia and fibula, inserting a metal plate, and sort of lining the bones up better to alter the stress patterns. Dr. Upandcomer did say, when I asked him, that no randomized trials had been done yet, but he was pretty sure it worked because he'd seen lots of patients do well.

I assume that Dr. McRae felt the same way about his operation thirty years ago; so I am a little fussy about evidence. Anyway, Dr. Upandcomer's plan didn't sound like a good idea to me, partly because the picture of all the hardware—screws, plates, and things—that that new procedure would leave in my knee seemed to me to make it potentially harder to put a new knee prosthesis into the knee when it came time for that later on. The wedge was just palliative—just temporizing. It was just a simple thought—all those screws seemed to me like they might get in the way. Anyway, I already had a screw.

A little while later, I went to see a different surgeon, who friends told me was sort of "Dr. Knee" in a particular city—a knee-man's knee-man. I wanted to know what he thought; if I should have that wedge operation, or what. So, I asked him. To get the picture, you need to see the set-up in your mind's eye—there was me sitting on a table, Dr. Knee facing me, and behind Dr. Knee, out of his line of sight, but in mine, was Dr. Knee's senior fellow, who, it happened, had actually trained with Dr. Upandcomer, the one who recommended the operation with the plates and screws.

Dr. Knee said that *he* thought that, if Dr. Upandcomer thought the new procedure would help me, I should have it.

I asked Dr. Knee, "Wouldn't the wedge surgery now make knee replacement later on much harder, with all those plates and screws in my knee?"

"Not at all," said Dr. Knee, shaking his head. But, just then I noticed that the senior fellow behind him was waving his arms at me trying to get my attention and silently mouthing the words, "Yes, it would," and nodding his head up and down. Dr. Knee turned around, and, like a scene on *Saturday Night Live*, the fellow suddenly stopped his waving and acted like he was just smoothing his hair down.

When you answer my RFP, please tell me why that wouldn't happen in your hospital. How do you make sure that, if the housekeeper or student nurse in my operating room sees something that could help me—maybe even save my life—he or she will speak up loudly, promptly, and directly and that the surgeon will praise that participation, not scowl. Explain to me how you make sure that the team really is a team, and that communication channels stay wide open, so that every patient—so that I—get the benefit of all the best information.

So, Spec 2A says "No needless pain—don't give me needless pain by doing things that don't help," and Spec 2B says, "Don't give me needless pain by the converse defect—failing to do things for me reliably and consistently that do help."

Spec 2C is a special case of the other two. It reads, "Relieve my pain." I'm stoic, but I'm not a Zen master. If it hurts, I want you to take the hurt away. That includes physical pain and emotional pain. I want you to relieve both.

Physical pain you can get right by using the science. I already know that from my own pain-free operations number three and number four. These were done with world-class pain control, and I'm going to tell you where, because you should know: Virginia Mason Clinic in Seattle, Washington, where I went for those procedures. Not a single moment of any pain at all, at any time. It wowed me.

And, it made me even more upset about the gaps our nation has in pain control. A few years ago, my hero, Joanne Lynn, led an IHI Collaborative on end-of-life care that focused on pain control. When we started, we found that cancer patients in a major hospital who were admitted explicitly to relieve their pain waited on average 110 minutes for their first dose of pain medicine.

Thanks to good science, we know how to relieve pain safely. I want you to promise me that you will use that knowledge, so that I do not suffer if I don't have to. No needless pain.

Emotional pain is more subtle. We all have our own version. My emotional pain gets worse when I'm alone, when I want to know something but no one will answer me, when I feel criticized or like someone thinks I'm stupid, when I'm frightened. So, your reply to my RFP will have to tell me how you plan to help me with that stuff. Will you promise me that I won't be separated from the people who love me? I won't hire any place that doesn't let my wife and kids into the ICU, recovery room, or emergency department any time I want them there. Any time. Will you promise me straight answers to my questions, and will you stick with me until I finally understand your answers?

You can see how this works at Terry Clemmer's ICU at LDS Hospital, which has open visitation and the best approach to helping family members I have seen anywhere. You can study it now at Geisinger Clinic in Pennsylvania, where Karen McKinley has been leading her medical ICU, though not yet the surgical ICU, to fully open visiting hours.

Specification Number Three Is "No Helplessness"

I can maybe show you this one better than talking about it.

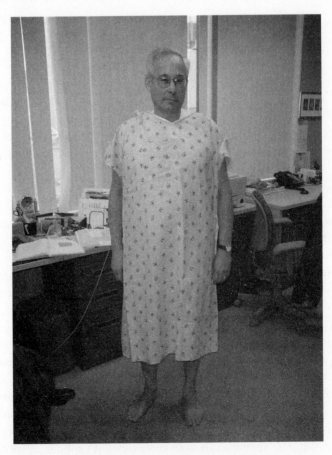

Berwick in a Hospital Gown

So you're laughing. Why are you laughing? Because I look ridiculous. It's a slippery slope from here to helplessness. I *do* look ridiculous —childlike, undignified, vulnerable. That's what I mean, partly, by helplessness. Look how much you can take away from me when I agree to become your patient. You can take away my clothes, my privacy, my right not to be naked. You can put things in my body orifices and veins. You can take away my pills, and give me yours. You can harm me with an error, and never tell me. You can read me your rules, but I cannot read you mine.

I'm looking for a place that won't let that happen. The two most important ways to prevent my helplessness are to share information with me and to give me choices. First, keep me posted. That'll begin with my medical record. No one can touch my knee who won't give me my medical record to read anytime I want it, no questions asked, and no delays. Better yet, let me keep my record with me, and I'll let you use it anytime you want.

To keep me from feeling helpless, you'll need to leave choices in my hands. You'll need to find out the way I want things, and adapt to me. You'll need to read my rules, and not just read me yours.

A close relative of mine was in a hospital this summer for a serious illness. She needed anticoagulation and blood tests every six hours. She also needed her blood chemistries monitored every six hours with a different blood test. Problem was, the orders were put in at separate times, and the six-hour intervals weren't synchronized. That meant my cousin had eight blood draws a day instead of four.

So, I asked on her behalf that they synchronize the blood drawing, but the IV nurse refused "because the doctor ordered it that way." So did the floor nurse, who looked pretty annoyed at me. They called the surgical resident, and he looked even more annoyed. He said that he refused to take responsibility for any risks that delaying one or the other of the blood tests would involve. My cousin was so scared that she cried. Moreover, he told us that this meant that at 2:00 a.m., he, not the IV nurse, would have to draw the blood.

That's what I mean about helplessness. Eight needle sticks when it could have been only four. Blaming the patient and her difficult relative for asking that a moronic scheduling defect be repaired. Shifting the burden to the patient. Treating an honest, logical request as a bother.

I'll tell you what I'd like. Tell me how you treat "patient's orders"— mine—as respectfully and carefully as you treat "doctor's orders," and maybe I'll let you get into my knee. If your feeling is that that makes me a "difficult patient," then save us both time and don't submit a proposal.

I guess I'd like an appendix to your application that tells me how you make sure that all of your staff understand that—that you hire people who have the attitude "The patient is the boss," and that you give them the tools to make it so.

If I'm not going to feel helpless, then I need to be able to reach you later on—after I go home—maybe months later, maybe even years later—with questions and suggestions. You make me helpless when you leave me confused with no way to get unconfused. I'd really appreciate 24/7 answers, if you can arrange that. Email access to the doctor would work just fine for me. Who knows when I might feel worried? If you tend to view discharge as "out of sight, out of mind," I don't think you can get the job. My knee—or the metal one you put into me—is hopefully going to be around for quite a while—twenty years, maybe, so I want you to remember me . . . that long.

It is interesting to me, and sad, that the surgeon who first did the wrong operation never, ever, called me or followed up on me in any way at all to see how I was doing, which has at least a little to do with how he is doing. How can he learn about the long run? Did he think I was done with my knee when he was? I'll give you extra points if you have a total knee registry, and use it a lot. Even more points if you follow up patients regularly for years, to understand the effects of your work on them over time.

Specification Number Four Is "No Unwanted Waiting"

This is sort of obvious. I want you to tell me how you prevent delays of all types. I am really busy, just like you are, and for most things, the best wait for me is no wait at all. In your clinics, I'd appreciate your using the Advanced Access model of Mark Murray and Catherine Tantau, like the Alaska Native Medical Center, and Luther Midelfort, and ThedaCare do, or like Everett Clinic or the Veterans Health Administration, so I can get an appointment any day I want it. In your hospital, I'd appreciate it if you'd use the brilliant work of Professor Eugene Litvak on how to smooth flow through your system. Maybe you could participate in IHI's Flow Collaboratives. That way, you won't leave me alone on gurneys in your hallway. You'll start my surgical case when you say you will. If you do a test, you'll store and retrieve it on demand, and if someone else already did the same test, you'll use that test instead of repeating it. You'll schedule my discharge in advance to the half-hour, and I won't have to wait around for a missing doctor's signature or because my medications haven't arrived.

I am already helping you with this one. In my bedroom closet, behind the sweaters, is my X-ray file. It contains almost all of the X-rays, MRIs, and CAT scans taken of my right knee in the past decade. Some are copies. Most are stolen. It's a complete file. It's probably also a felony.

Why am I a felon? Well, let's review the history. Since 1991, I have received surgery, care, or opinions for my knee in seven different locations—six in New England and one on the West Coast—from eleven physicians and surgeons, four physical therapists, and a masseur. I have had eight different X-ray, MRI, and CAT scan sessions in five different facilities. On no occasion at all did anyone who saw me have anyone else's X-rays or images to look at—only their own—except when I, myself, physically transported them. This required me to take time, over and over again, traveling to hospital file rooms, filling out forms, and waiting while they searched. On two occasions, when I tried to borrow films to transport them, the facility told me they were lost.

So, I figured, why not lose them to me? They're no more lost than they were before, except now at least one person knows exactly where they are lost to.

Since I became a felon, every single clinician I have seen about my knee has had every single image that was ever done in the past ten years. The Berwick right knee imaging retrieval system has become 100 percent reliable. And, the delays waiting for people to find or fetch films have fallen quite low—to zero, as a matter of fact. Well, my closet is a little messy, so it can take me a few seconds.

Just a warning: to the young people in the audience, I am not advising you to steal your own X-rays and medical records so as to improve reliability, decrease helplessness, and drive delays to zero while also saving hospitals and clinics the costs and delays of retrieval and tracking down lost items. That would not make any sense, would it?

Do you know that in the Military Health Command, patients can store and carry their own medical records?

Specification Number Five Is "No Waste"

Now, do I really care about that one? After all, my health insurance is pretty good, and, if you want to raise your costs by creating scrap or wasting materials or duplicating efforts, isn't that your problem, not mine?

Of course, the good citizen in me wants you to reduce your costs by reducing your waste. European health care systems, after all, tick away at one-half the cost of ours. Here are some recent figures: the OECD

[Organisation for Economic Co-operation and Development] nations provide comprehensive, universal health care at $2,000 per person per year, while we spend $4,800 in the United States. I am astounded by the myths chiseled into concrete in the minds of Americans about these differences. The myth that people flock to us for care they cannot get in Canada or England. The myth that these other systems are disciplined by rationing that we don't accept.

The myths are wrong, and it is one of the greatest frustrations I have as a student of improvement that I cannot seem ever to win the attention or curiosity of American health care leaders to study and harvest bold, new ideas from these non-US systems. The answers we need for America's health care do not lie in our normal experience. They lie outside our normal experience. The knee surgery outcomes in Sweden are good. I think they're better than ours. I know that their postoperative care is more integrated than ours. I know that they have a national knee arthroplasty registry with over seventy thousand entries in it. In your response to my RFP, maybe you'd like to tell me how you are learning from other nations about how to make better care with less money. If you answer that question, you may be the only one who does.

But, actually, my knee and I have a more selfish reason to ask you about waste. It relates to something Paul O'Neill first told me: the importance of what he calls "a habit of excellence." He thinks, and I agree, that excellence in a system, to be reliable, can't be divisible. You can't say, "Be excellent here, but it's okay to be sloppy there."

Waste is a symptom of a defective process. It is non-excellence. I want my knee in the hands of people and a place who are intolerant of the disorder, duplication, unpredictability, and inattention to detail that lie at the root of waste, because then I can predict with more confidence that my care may be orderly, coordinated, anticipatory, and attentive. I want my care from a place where a habit of excellence creates a sheen and leanness, a sensitivity in real time, a calmness and steadiness that no glutton seeks or understands.

I've got to tell you that, when I finally read my whole RFP, overall, I got nervous. It's really asking for a lot, and it is very self-centered. It leaves me with two big questions. First, does anyone want to answer it? And, second, *can* anyone answer it?

I just can't help you with the first question, "Do you want to pay attention to me?" I can't make anyone want to serve me. That's your call, not mine. If I ever could actually issue an RFP, and take my money with me to a winning applicant, I'd do it. With one shot left between me and cross-country skiing, I've just got to take the best shot.

But you and I both know that I can't do that. I can't really shop, not much. Health care is a niche market, and my choices are very, very limited. In fact, the only thing more limited than my choices is the information on the basis of which I would choose, if I could choose.

That's changing. I hope it'll change fast. Transparency about results seems more and more important to me as I age and as my bone-on-bone wears away. I was interested that, even though nobody made them do it, John Toussaint at ThedaCare and colleagues in eight organizations in Wisconsin have taken it upon themselves to publish their own performance data, warts and all, on a whole bunch of indicators, and more over time, as part of the Wisconsin Collaborative for Healthcare Quality. I applaud them. That's one of the places in the country where I actually could make some choices on the things I care about. I just wish I could do that for my knee.

So, I'll have to turn to my second question, "Is this fantasy or can it be done? If anyone did want to try to meet my specs, could they?" Here, the answer is easier; it's "Yes." Nothing in my RFP, nothing at all, is out of reach. For almost every detail, I know a supplier right now. I can avoid surgical infections if I go to Intermountain Health Care. I can avoid ventilator-associated pneumonia if I go to Dominican Hospital in Santa Cruz. My indwelling IV won't get infected at Baptist DeSoto Hospital. My wife and kids can visit me any time, day or night, in the medical ICU at Geisinger Clinic. If I were cared for in the Military Health Command, I could carry my own medical record, and I could read it anytime I want. I might have no pain at all—I did have no pain at all—at Virginia Mason. My primary care delays would be zero because of open access schedules at Luther Midelfort or ThedaCare, and my specialty delays would be constantly falling at Alaska Native Medical Center in Anchorage. I could wear my street clothes in a Planetree Unit, and get to my doctors through email anytime at Group Health Cooperative of Puget Sound. At Ekjö Hospital in Jönköping County, Sweden, the costs of my care would be 40 percent of the US costs, with the same outcomes, lower complications, and more coordinated rehabilitation. My care would be integrated across inpatient and outpatient settings by an electronic medical record in the VA, and digital radiology in the Indian Health Service would allow me to clean out my closet.

In ten years of hard work, we have all together brought health care from the state of having no cloth to the state of having no quilt. The patches are made. The stitching is the problem. Look around you; almost everyone in this room has a piece of the answer. I could have exactly what I want if I could cut myself into pieces. I'd get my respirator care at Dominican, my IV line at Baptist DeSoto, my medical record at the Washington Medical Center, my pain control in Seattle, and my appointments in Anchorage. I'd have the transparency of the Wisconsin Collaborative, the respectfulness of Planetree, the orderliness and sparseness of Jönköping, the teamwork and nursing morale of Hackensack and North Shore–Long Island Jewish, the flow management of Mayo Clinic in Rochester, Minnesota, and the email system of Dr. Gordon Moore in Rochester, New York, or Dr. Chuck Kilo in Portland, Oregon. I see what I want and need; it's just scattered all around.

Someone, please, now put it together. I need a quilt, not patches. This isn't just a speech for me. This is real. It will be dark one night, and your nurses will be tiptoeing outside my room. And I will be lying there, in the bed you make for me, scared and wondering: Am I safe? Will I die here? Will I ski again? Where is my wife? What are you thinking? Do you know I am here? Do you know my name? Do you know my name?

Do it right—for me or for anyone. No needless death, no needless pain, no helplessness, no unwanted waiting, no waste. Don't do it just for me . . . no, wait a minute—do it just for me.

Our theme for this National Forum is "courage." What does this have to do with courage? It's only a knee. Just a knee. Thank God. It could be my heart. It could be cancer. It could be ALS, or a disabling psychosis. It could be pain for years, not hours, or losing the ability to speak, or see, or reason, not just to ski the moguls. I could be, not an American with a bad knee, but a Thai with dengue or an African with AIDS.

There's the courage: to see myself in others. What if they're just like me? What if everyone I want to help is just me, in disguise? Tomorrow, Forum keynote speaker Paul Farmer will talk to us about some of the poorest people in the world—in rural Haiti. What if they're just like us? What if every one of them, whether we ask them or not, has an RFP, too, as complex, as poetic, and every bit as important to him or her, as mine is to me, or as yours is to you?

The great Gandhi sat with a child, and said, "I, too, have felt what I am asking you to feel." Then, and not before, he was able to help. We are no Gandhis, but I am coming to believe that we cannot relieve the pain of others until we feel our own. It is the only sustainable source of sufficient will for change. We will help them with what they need when we know what we need. We will honor and respect their wishes when we have trusted and respected our own.

Imagine the care you'll need before the Red Sox finally win. You couldn't be in a better place to search for it—four thousand strong at this Forum, four thousand more joining by satellite—a movement well begun, waiting to help. Wish for what you need, trust what you wish for, and then promise no less to the people you serve. If we can have the courage to see it that way, then, I promise you, we'll sweep the Series— clean sweep. Red Sox, eat your hearts out.

FURTHER READING

Fisher ES, Wennberg DE, Stukel TA, Gottlieb DJ, Lucas FL, Pinder EL. The implications of regional variations in Medicare spending. Part 1: The content, quality, and accessibility of care. *Ann Intern Med.* 2003 Feb 18;138(4):273–287.

Fisher ES, Wennberg DE, Stukel TA, Gottlieb DJ, Lucas FL, Pinder EL. The implications of regional variations in Medicare spending. Part 2: Health outcomes and satisfaction with care. *Ann Intern Med.* 2003 Feb 18;138(4):288–298.

Chapter 2

SOME IS NOT A NUMBER, SOON IS NOT A TIME

COMMENTARY

C. Joseph McCannon

WHEN DON BERWICK took the stage to deliver this keynote speech on December 14, 2004, I was standing off to his right in the massive ballroom at the Marriott World Center in Orlando. Though the crowd was buzzing with excitement, I was feeling anxious.

What he was about to announce was fraught with risk—to the Institute for Healthcare Improvement (IHI), to the health care industry, to Don, and to everyone involved in the enterprise. He was going to challenge us: avoid one hundred thousand unnecessary deaths in hospitals over the next eighteen months. In one move, he was asking us to admit our serious flaws and demanding that we take action to correct them.

It was boldness personified. It would make people uncomfortable. It would introduce complexity. It would court controversy. It would also be very hard to pull off, and that's what I was wrestling with behind the stage.

Less than a month earlier, Don asked me and a group of IHI colleagues to prepare this "Campaign" that would be unveiled at the National Forum. Together, we burned the midnight oil, generating materials, logos, literature reviews, and measurement strategies. We canvassed experts from across the country. We secured the support of major hospital systems and professional associations.

But with one week to go before launch, our small team was still unsure of itself. Wouldn't it be better, we reasoned, to have Don simply float the idea of a Campaign during his speech? If response was good, then we could start the Campaign a bit later, in April.

I was nominated to bestow our wisdom on Don. He listened patiently and then said, "We are going to launch this Campaign on December 14."

Thinking perhaps he hadn't heard me, I rephrased my argument.

He smiled and said again, "We are going to launch this Campaign on December 14."

I tried again. "But we won't be ready! We could create a furor! We could hurt our reputation! We could fail!"

To that, he simply said, "You cannot fail."

It was like a Zen koan. I didn't quite get it. I walked away, chastened, and told the team that we would need to redouble our efforts.

I was almost resigned as he launched into his Forum keynote speech. All I could do was listen. Thank goodness.

When he introduced the 100,000 Lives Campaign at the 2004 National Forum, Don acknowledged how accustomed we can become to expecting the worst, to accepting harm to patients as an unavoidable product of health care. He articulated all of the reasons why we could fail. He stated all of the objections in advance. And then he insisted that we had to do it anyway—that patients and families could not wait one more day, that our time had come. This is, above all, a speech about taking chances, about doing great things in our lives, about being courageous. It is—in some very essential way—the invitation that we have all been waiting for.

So many rose to the challenge in the months that followed. More than two thousand hospitals enrolled in the Campaign by June 2005 and thirty-one hundred would sign up by the Campaign's close one year later. Hundreds of hospitals demonstrated spectacular results, avoiding fatal deterioration or delivering highly reliable care for heart attacks, and becoming mentors to the rest of the nation. The initiative marked a national inflection point in reducing infections, driving down ventilator-associated pneumonias and central-line bacteremia, punctuated several years later by the spectacular work of Peter Pronovost in the state of Michigan.

Boards of directors stood in front of their communities and said, "We are harming people. We can do better." CEOs plastered the walls of their hospital lobbies with run charts showing their progress *and* their failures. Providers and patients—some of them victims of life-changing harm— gathered around tables to discuss how to redesign systems to be more reliable and more sensitive to their needs. It was remarkable to see.

Of course, just about every bad thing that Don predicted might happen did. Some doctors felt defensive. Some researchers challenged the evidence base for the interventions we introduced. Our measurement strategy became contentious, and a fascinating academic debate emerged over how much of the progress observed across the nation could be attributed directly to the Campaign. The media turned its attention to IHI (to the order of 250 million media impressions) and our small organization had to grow in ways that were challenging and sometimes painful.

What's more, the work is not done. Every year, hundreds of thousands of patients are still unintentionally harmed by the care they receive and, if anything, health care is growing more complex and dangerous.

But on that December day and in the eighteen months that followed, we took an important, bold step forward. An industry—and its expectations—changed forever.

No group felt the power of this Campaign more than the ten-person IHI team that started and ran it. We overcame our fear. We became close friends. We studied our progress every day and innovated constantly in response. We could not fail—we could only learn and improve.

Don Berwick pushed us off that cliff and, son of a gun, we flew.

SOME IS NOT A NUMBER, SOON IS NOT A TIME

PLENARY ADDRESS
INSTITUTE FOR HEALTHCARE IMPROVEMENT
16TH ANNUAL NATIONAL FORUM ON QUALITY
IMPROVEMENT IN HEALTH CARE
ORLANDO, FLORIDA, DECEMBER 14, 2004

IF YOU HAVEN'T heard . . . the Boston Red Sox did it. Eighty-six years after their last World Series championship, and twenty-six championships behind the New York Yankees, they came from three games behind in a best-of-seven league playoff against the Yankees, and won four straight games against the Yankees and then four straight against the St. Louis Cardinals.

I cried. Not because baseball is important, but because I remembered the night in 1986 when my two sons—Ben and Dan—and I were watching game six of the World Series—Red Sox versus the New York Mets—when, one out—one strike—away from winning—our team screwed up and, incredibly, lost. I remembered Ben—age ten—sobbing as he staggered upstairs to bed. In October 2004, Ben, Dan, and I were in separate cities—Boston, Washington, and Orlando—but we could just as well have been in the same room together, watching game four of the Series this time. We knew exactly what we were feeling together.

The next day in Boston a few drivers even slowed down to let other cars in front of them. In *Boston*! We locals call it "Red Sox Nation."

The downside is that I lost my bet from my speech at last year's National Forum. If you were there, you may remember that I asked, "Which will happen first—the health care system we need and deserve, or the Red Sox winning the series?" I bet against the Red Sox.

My mistake. I should have set a deadline for fixing health care.

I should have listened to my second son, Dan. Dan was a varsity player in the other great game of this American autumn—politics. Dan is twenty-six, and he is one of the nomadic young generation X-ers who run the incredibly complex campaign structures from election to election in our country. In four years since college, Dan has worked on campaigns in Virginia, Texas, Washington, D.C., Oregon, Wisconsin, Minnesota, New Mexico, Ohio, and Florida. A weekend's work for him could be arranging for an army of canvassers to knock on fifty thousand doors in a swing state.

So, I asked Dan to come to the IHI one day and meet with us to teach us how to mobilize—what a campaign really looks like. You see, I've been thinking. If we're not careful, I mean, at the rate we're going, the Red Sox may not just win one or two World Series before health care gets safe, effective, patient-centered, timely, efficient, and equitable, they'll beat the Yankees' total of twenty-six. In a campaign, you can't afford that patience. An election bears down on you like a truck on a highway. The clock is a tyrant. If you spend too much time getting ready, you'll lose.

Dan said that political campaigns have a golden rule, which gives me the title of this speech: "Some Is Not a Number, Soon Is Not a Time."

"Some is not a number, soon is not a time." When I heard him say that, the lights turned on.

Dan said that a campaign works with a single target—he called it "50 percent plus one"—that's the number of votes you need to win. Not one less. And, of course, it has a deadline—Election Day. Every step of a well-oiled campaign machine, every day of work against the ticking clock, has targets, too. It may be doors knocked on—thirty thousand this weekend—or phone calls completed—fifty thousand this week—or voters driven to the polls on Election Day. Dan calls these targets "the hard count." That means exactly what it sounds like. The tasks are specific, countable, scheduled. They're either done, or not done. Like Yoda said, "Do, or not do. There is no try." "Maybe" doesn't count. "Later" doesn't count. Some is not a number, soon is not a time. Rule One.

These are other rules. For example, the rule of simplification. Make the task simple.

Another rule is the same one Gloria Steinem told us at the National Forum when she was our keynote speaker in 2001. She said, in effect, "Make room for everyone." Meet each voter exactly where he or she is, and create one small, local step—the next step—that they can take toward you. It is graduated enrollment—read an email, send an email, send a dollar, send $10, send $500, work an evening for the candidate, and so on.

Another rule: Great campaigns stay on message: they have "message discipline." In fact, the idea of discipline infuses a good campaign—message discipline, the discipline of the hard count, the discipline of deadlines and schedules. "Some is not a number, soon is not a time" is discipline.

Oh, I wish you could have been in Boston at World Series time. It was intense. Out to dinner with friends, waiting on line for coffee, getting into a taxi, meeting a neighbor—it didn't matter where you were, you talked about the Red Sox. Our fingers crossed; we prepared our advice just in case the Red Sox manager happened to call and ask us if Derek Lowe should start or not. We didn't dare hope, but we couldn't stop hoping.

All that intensity. And about baseball! A pastime. A game.

I want that in our work . . . the work of improvement. Is it impossible to imagine that we wake up in the morning and rush to the papers to see the box score on our game—the one we're *playing*, not the one we're just *watching*?

I'm losing my patience. Maybe it's my age. Maybe it's my emails from people who keep telling me what went wrong with their care. Maybe it's the words of Honor Page, who spoke at our Forum last year, the mother of Annie, who has cystic fibrosis. When I asked her what she would most want health care leaders to hear, Honor said to me, "Tell them the clock is ticking for Annie."

Or, maybe it's the hope that I find in the amazing results that many of you in this room are getting every day now from your work to improve care. You're doing so much so well; you're putting actual transformation within our reach. Now, we need to grab it. I'm losing my patience.

So, here is what I think we should do. I think we should save one hundred thousand lives. And I think we should do that by June 14, 2006—eighteen months from today. Some is not a number, soon is not a time. Here's the number: one hundred thousand. Here's the time: June 14, 2006—9:00 a.m.

The Red Sox did their job, now let's do ours. Now let's do ours. I think the time for discipline has arrived—the time for getting the job done.

This is going to be it: one hundred thousand lives; June 14, 2006.

We're going to do it with a Campaign—a world-class Campaign. We are going to elect quality. Our plan, for a "100,000 Lives Campaign," has been revised and led by a fantastic team at the IHI—in fact we're almost all involved—but especially Jessica Berwick, David Calkins, Sharon Eloranta, Don Goldmann, Joelle Grande, Andy Hackbarth, Madge Kaplan, Bob Lloyd, Joe McCannon, Alexi Nazem, Jane Roessner, Lindsay Ruhlmann, and Jonathan Small. A lot of what follows now is based on the design sketched by that amazing team. I can't thank them enough.

The theme of this Forum is, "How?" It comes directly from a poignant email I got last year from a Forum participant who wrote, basically, this: "I get it. I get it. You do not have to tell me one more time how bad health care quality is, or how much better we can be. You don't have to tell me one more time what to accomplish. I know the 'what.' What I need now is the 'how.'"

One hundred thousand lives; June 14, 2006. That's the "what." Now: the "how" . . .

Here's how we're going to do it. We're going to take some things we know about life-saving changes in care systems and processes and make them our standards—national standards. We're going to harness what we know—everywhere.

We know a ton. You in this very room have found dozens of life-saving, life-extending improvements in many of your hospitals. IHI's annual progress report celebrates twenty-two organizations that have turned promising ideas into action—and I know you'll enjoy reading about their successes. We will convert their success into our platform. On your chairs right now are some materials that describe the six interventions—the "hows"—that are at the heart of the 100,000 Lives Campaign. They'll be the route to success. Where I am going is this: to ask that we get these changes—all of them—into sixteen hundred American hospitals within the next year. The six changes are these:

- *Rapid Response Teams* to intercept unexpected deterioration of inpatients
- Reliable, evidence-based care for *acute myocardial infarction* (heart attacks) to reduce mortality rates
- Use of the so-called *Ventilator Bundle,* a set of scientifically validated processes used for management of ventilated patients to help prevent ventilator-acquired pneumonia
- Use of the *Central Line Bundle,* to keep indwelling central venous catheters from becoming infected

- Prevention of *surgical site infections*, largely by reliable use of appropriately chosen and appropriately timed perioperative antibiotics
- Prevention of severe *adverse drug events*, largely through the use of so-called medication reconciliation procedures

Let's take a more detailed look. First, Rapid Response Teams. These teams are called Medical Emergency Teams in the original Australian experimental literature. Hospitals create these teams to respond immediately to clinicians—usually nurses—who are getting worried about a particular inpatient, often with only a gut feel. Something seems to be going wrong with Mrs. Smith, even if they can't put their finger on it. In the usual system, these worries can lie there, unresolved, not responded to, for a long time—a day or two, or more. Meanwhile, too often, Mrs. Smith slips into worse and worse shape, sort of under our noses. An urgent clinical response happens finally only when disaster strikes—her heart stops, a code call, Code Blue. Rapid Response Teams come sooner. They come to Mrs. Smith's bedside when someone gets worried because someone gets worried. A nurse or other clinician can call them on his or her own initiative, without asking permission from, say, an admitting physician up front. The Rapid Response Team comes right away—Code Gray—assesses the patient urgently, forms an impression, makes a plan. They're trying to prevent the disaster that might have occurred later on—hours or days later. Often, they do.

How good is it? In published trials, in Australia, Rapid Response Teams had a stunning effect on outcomes. Deaths fell; so did code calls. In the seminal article, published in the *Medical Journal of Australia*, the authors reported a 27 percent decline in hospital mortality rates with this single intervention, alone.

Rapid Response Teams were picked up by some American hospitals, and the IHI has been trying them with a number of our Pursuing Perfection and IMPACT network hospitals. Now, some of those hospitals have found effects on code calls and unanticipated deaths just as good as in the Australian reports. The Society for Critical Care Medicine has endorsed this change. Rapid Response Teams are life saving and feasible. But, they aren't at all yet the norm. Most hospitals don't have them. Because of our Campaign, they will. So, people who might have died won't.

The same is true for the second intervention we're promoting: what we in the IHI call "reliable" care for acute myocardial infarction—heart attacks—AMI. In the IHI, we've become very interested in reliability. Its definition is a little squirrelly, but, for our purposes here, reliability means just the number of times something is done correctly divided by the number of times it was tried. For example, if, for every hundred AMI patients that we intended to give beta-blockers to, ninety actually got the drug, then the reliability is 90 divided by 100, or 90 percent.

We can up the stakes on reliability by bundling together a set of things that ought to happen. Take AMI, again. Let's say that we've decided that suitable AMI victims in our hospital ought to get seven specific interventions: early administration of beta-blockers and aspirin, beta-blockers and aspirin at discharge, an ACE inhibitor or angiotensin-receptor blocker at discharge if they have systolic dysfunction, timely reperfusion, and smoking cessation counseling. Most doctors and nurses would endorse these because of strong, scientific evidence. Now, we could score our reliability as a list of numbers—one score per item—say 90 percent for beta-blockers at admission, 95 percent for aspirin at discharge, 83 percent for timely reperfusion, and so on. That's a standard way to do it. But, if we want to be really tough, we can score ourselves on a sort of pass-fail basis for the whole bundle of things—a patient gets a "yes" if we actually did everything we planned to do, and a "no" if anything, even one thing, was left out. We in the IHI call this bundled scoring system "raising the bar" on performance.

In health care right now, we are mostly reporting reliabilities in AMI care of components—each separate step—and good places are scoring, say, 90 percent to 95 percent. Today, 95 percent on each AMI indicator would earn you a pretty good score from Medicare or your QIO [Quality Improvement Organization]. If we take the tougher look—the "all-or-nothing" look—the reliabilities fall pretty fast—probably to well below 50 percent for most AMI care. Here is how it looks for another reliability issue: proper initial treatment of community-acquired pneumonia, as described in the 2004 National Healthcare Quality Report from the Agency for Healthcare Research and Quality. (AHRQ has chosen this Forum as a place to unveil this year's report.)

A few players with the IHI—again in Pursuing Perfection and IMPACT—have been trying to change that game. They are trying to get highly reliable on the total package of AMI care—the whole package. To do this, they have to make many changes, like using standard protocols for care, providing reminder systems, and changing job designs, to ensure that the right drugs and procedures are used absolutely every time they should be.

Here is what happens when they do that. At Hackensack University Hospital and McLeod Regional Medical Center, working on reliable

AMI care has cut inpatient AMI mortality rates in half in less than a year—from the US average of about 10 percent down to 6 percent or 5 percent. In the IHI we refer to the order of magnitude of the defects in care. If we are getting it right all but one time in ten approximately, then our defect rate—our rate of unreliability—is one over ten, which is "ten to the minus one" power [10^{-1}]. If we are able to reduce defects to one part per one hundred, then our unreliability is an order of magnitude better—"ten to the minus two" power [10^{-2}], or one over one hundred. What McLeod, Hackensack, and others are doing is rejecting satisfaction with "ten to the minus one" performance; and aiming for "ten to the minus two," which cuts AMI deaths about in half.

The third intervention we're proposing is what we call the Ventilator Bundle—for the management of people on respirator machines—ventilators—especially in intensive care units. People on these machines can get pneumonias from them—ventilator-associated pneumonias [VAP]—and these can be killers. The CDC offers guidelines on preventing VAP, but, just as with AMI care, reliability in adherence to these guidelines is only in "ten to the minus one" range. For bundles of standards, it's much lower.

IHI has an intensive care unit redesign team, which brought together experts from the Society for Critical Care Medicine and from European societies to try to define a scientifically grounded "bundle" of rules for care of patients on ventilators, and they came up with the Ventilator Bundle with five elements: elevation of the head of the bed by 30 to 45 degrees, peptic ulcer prophylaxis, deep venous thrombosis prophylaxis, so-called "sedation vacations" lightening sedative use daily, and daily assessment of readiness for extubation. Hospitals that have managed to get to "ten to the minus two" reliability for this Ventilator Bundle are now reporting dramatic—unprecedented—reductions in VAP. Dominican Santa Cruz Hospital and Baptist Hospital in Southaven, Mississippi, have gone month after month—sometimes nearly an entire year—without a single case of VAP.

Intervention number four, reducing central venous line (CVL) infections, like number three, uses a bundle of proven interventions. Without them, CVL infections can kill thousands of patients each year. Using the Central Line Bundle reliably at Baptist DeSoto has nearly eliminated these infections. Dr. Rick Shannon, at Allegheny Hospital in Pittsburgh, has gotten the same results.

Our fifth target for "ten to the minus two" reliability is in prophylaxis against surgical site infections—SSI prevention. Here, the main clinical challenge is to prescribe and administer the correct perioperative antibiotics for the proper cases within a strict time window surrounding the time of incision. It's not the only thing, but it's the main thing. Most hospitals—most good hospitals—hit the window at "ten to the minus one" levels of reliability. Great ones—hospitals that just won't accept that risk and morbidity any longer—are developing work flows, standard order sets, and clinical cultures that ensure parts-per-hundred reliability in antibiotic timing at a minimum. The SSI interventions also include avoidance of shaving of surgical sites and strict perioperative blood sugar control. Mercy Health Center in Oklahoma City has seen a steady increase in the number of surgical cases between successive infections—up to 401, but now that number has grown to 879 without a single SSI in targeted cases—not one yet. Yankees, eat your hearts out!

Finally, the Campaign's sixth arena of life-saving process change, adverse drug event (ADE) prevention, has to do with medication errors—the cause of almost one-fifth of the forty-four thousand to ninety-eight thousand deaths in American hospitals each year associated with avoidable injuries from care. One particularly powerful way to cut down on bad medication errors, and the one change we will concentrate on first in our Campaign to reduce ADEs, is to use reconciliation procedures at transfer. Right now patients are vulnerable to medication mix-ups because of the lack of coordination and continuity between outpatient and inpatient care. Clinical office practices and hospitals that treat a patient's list of prescribed medicines as a critical piece of medical information that must constantly match up and move between settings are taking an enormous step toward preventing harm. The Joint Commission is now putting medication reconciliation into its safety standards, and our Campaign will spread that change into thousands of hospitals.

Now, let me ask what proportion of American hospitals routinely use—correctly use—any or all of these six innovations in care: Rapid Response Teams, "ten to the minus two" reliability for bundles of scientifically correct care for AMIs, ventilator management, and surgical site infection prevention, correct procedures for elimination of central line infections, and medication reconciliation?

Second, if all hospitals did all six, how many deaths in hospitals would be eliminated or delayed?

Let's do some figuring. . . .

Well, the Australians reported a 27 percent decline in hospital deaths with their Rapid Response Teams, and a number of American hospitals are now repeating that experience pretty closely. Let's say that we're not nearly as good as the Australians. Let's say that our Rapid Response Teams can reduce deaths in hospitals by 10 percent—less than half the success experienced by the pioneers. An average five-hundred-bed hospital would have about forty thousand admissions a year, and, say, a raw mortality rate of 3 percent. That's twelve hundred deaths a year. Cut that by 10 percent, and Rapid Response Teams would save something like 120 lives per year, or roughly one life for every four beds per year.

If we can believe the experience of Hackensack and McLeod, then high reliability in care of heart attacks appears to cut AMI death rates about in half. If, say, 2.5 percent of the admissions to our hypothetical five-hundred-bed hospital are AMIs—one thousand admissions, and the initial death rate of 10 percent falls to 5 percent, then deaths each year would fall from one hundred to fifty, a saving of fifty lives.

For an average five-hundred-bed hospital, an 80 percent reduction in ventilator-associated pneumonias and lethal drug errors would each delay or prevent ten deaths per year; and an 80 percent reduction in surgical site infections would prevent about thirty deaths. Proper prevention of central line infections could avoid another ten deaths.

The total: with six changes in care, 230 lives saved per year in a five-hundred-bed hospital—just shy of one life per year for every two beds. But, maybe that's too optimistic. After all, changes in the real world don't always pan out as they did in published trials. So, to be conservative, let's cut the figure, say, about in half. Let's say, not 230, but 125 lives per year in a five-hundred-bed hospital—one life for every four beds. Remember, that's only half the gains that published papers and known improvement projects in real settings have found.

If that's our estimate, then to prevent, or at least to delay, one hundred thousand deaths, we would need to change these six processes for a total of about four hundred thousand beds. Some is not a number. There are the numbers: six changes, four hundred thousand. That's the hard count.

How about start now? Soon is not a time.

Campaigns have field operations. So do we. Their job is to figure out where the voters are, which doors to knock on to get out the vote. So, we have our hard count: four hundred thousand beds—where are they? Well, taking an average hospital size of about two hundred and fifty beds—not unrealistic—that means we need sixteen hundred hospitals. Our Campaign has to find sixteen hundred hospitals, one-third of American hospitals, to sign up. If they are smaller, we'll need more—maybe two thousand. Our field operation has to reach something like that—sixteen hundred to two thousand American hospitals.

Campaigns have careful messaging and communications—message discipline. So must we. My email buddy says, "Enough of 'what'! Tell me 'how.'" Our Campaign has to get the "how" right, linked to the "what." We would need to link those messages to help when and where help is needed. As with voters, we'll need to meet each hospital on its own terms, and help it find exactly the next step it can feasibly take—not too big, but in the right direction. If six changes are too many, how about three? How about one? Welcome, everybody. What would you like to do to help?

Motivation will count. One specific motivational and educational resource I want to mention as a brief detour is a series of seven videos supported by the Robert Wood Johnson Foundation and based on the many lessons we've learned so far in the Pursuing Perfection initiative. IHI is making them available for the first time starting at this Forum. Frank Christopher and Matthew Eisen, the producers of this series, will be leading a premier showing of the introductory video tomorrow morning in a breakfast session. I encourage you to attend.

We can save one hundred thousand lives in American hospitals per year if we can get sixteen hundred hospitals—maybe fewer—to make six changes in their care. To do it by June 14, 2006, they'll need some help.

My mentor and inspiration, Sister Mary Jean Ryan, gave me this quotation [by Christopher Logue], which I love:

> Come to the edge.
> We might fall.
> Come to the edge.
> It's too high!
> COME TO THE EDGE!
> And they came
> And he pushed
> And they flew.

> Used with permission.
> © Christopher Logue, "Come to the Edge, 1996."

I can guess what you're thinking. You probably have some problems with this plan. Let me guess.

When I was a small child, we read in school a newspaper for kids called, *My Weekly Reader*. On the back page of every issue was a drawing under a heading that said, "What's wrong with this picture?" The game was to find the eight or ten goofs in the drawing—the horse had five legs, or, in those days, the father was doing dishes instead of the mother.

Today, we call this "failure modes and effects analysis."

Let's play, "What's wrong with this picture?" Here I am, drunk on the Red Sox win, saying we can save one hundred thousand lives in the next eighteen months. Obviously, we can't. Where did I go wrong? Find seven things wrong with this picture.

Wrong Thing One: The changes won't work. These alleged results, reported anecdotally or in nonrandomized studies, aren't valid or replicable. Confounding secular trends—innovations in drugs or better materials—are masquerading as the effects of reliability.

Well, maybe. But, in the packets on your chairs and on the IHI's website, www.ihi.org, you can find the fully referenced literature—journal papers, studies, meta-analyses, and review papers. They provide some of the evidence for the six proposed changes. We've also given you the storyboards, and even contact names, for the organizations that have tried these changes and reported back their results. You be the judge. Check the data, check the reports, and see what level of confidence these build in you. Enough, maybe, to start, and see?

Wrong Thing Two: You're already doing it. You've had internal response teams for a decade. Your AMI care is the best in your region. You always give perioperative antibiotics on time.

If so, good for you. Maybe you don't need to be one of the hospitals our Campaign has to target. You're already there. But, one minor request: please check. Check your own data. If you have Rapid Response Teams, are they used? Are they properly designed and supported? Is your AMI care reliable truly at parts per hundred? Or, have you excelled within the envelope of usual performance—only parts per ten? Which ways do you keep score—for composites—bundles? Or for components? Are you raising the bar, or merely at the bar? And, what would happen to deaths—how many lives hang in the balance of that choice between reliable parts and a reliable whole?

I must say, if, in the end, you're sure you're there—already at the destination we want for the sixteen hundred hospitals, we really need your help. You can be a mentor. You can be a precinct captain. Maybe you can take on a whole state. McLeod has not stopped at trying to raise the bar for itself. McLeod is actually training many of the hospitals in its region—even its competitors—on how to improve the reliability of their AMI care. Maybe the lives you can save are in a hospital other than your own. Join our Campaign staff. Take on five hospitals that surround you, with one thousand beds, and save, say, 250 lives next year that way.

I really do want to acknowledge that every one of you in this room is already working hard on improving patient care—really hard. You've already got your work cut out for you in the months ahead and now we're asking you to take on something more—and to get results even faster. Well, this might be pretty annoying, but, yes, it's true. This Campaign raises expectations of all of us. And we're doing so because your good work so far tells us that we can get those results. It will help with some of your external compliance issues. A lot of our Campaign changes overlap with current and future requirements of organizations whose standards you will want to pay attention to: CMS, JCAHO, and others. This Campaign can be a "twofer."

Wrong Thing Three: We can't get the data. A lot of hospitals can't track their own mortality rates, and not many can adjust those measurements properly for case mix. It may be impossible, or nearly so, to keep score. We can talk glibly about "hard counts," but counting may prove harder than you think.

It is not impossible. Our Campaign is going to help you, and us, to keep track of our progress in more ways than one—four ways for starters. First, we'll simply keep count of the number of hospitals—and the total beds—that agree to commit themselves to these changes. We'll count sign-ups. Second, we'll ask participating hospitals to keep track of and report in on the process changes they make. Who has put Rapid Response Teams into place? Who has instituted the Ventilator Bundle? Whose AMI care is at ten to the minus two? Adding up process changes will allow us to model and estimate the effects on lives saved. Third, for hospitals that are willing, and maybe for a random sample, we will offer guidance on how actually to measure local mortality rates, and, if you wish, to report your gains like many members of IHI's IMPACT network are already doing. Fourth, using the brilliant work of Professor Brian Jarman, we will be working with CMS and the MedPar database to follow hospital standardized mortality rates in participating hospitals as a group—essentially tracking mortality rates over time.

That's not all, by any means. Our Campaign will be dynamic. You'll help us, and together we'll get better and better in the months ahead both in refining our change packages and measuring our successes.

Remember that measurement is a bit easier in our Campaign because the changes we seek aren't small—they are big; and this works in our favor in sorting signal from noise. Borgess Hospital in Kalamazoo had pretty good grounds for claiming one hundred lives saved, or so, and the run chart at Baptist DeSoto—a two-hundred-bed facility—leaves little doubt about the effects of their work on reliability in ICU care.

Wrong Thing Four: You'll get roasted in the press, and filleted in court. After all, any journalist worth her salt, told that you will now prevent one hundred thousand deaths, will tee up a first question like, "Do you mean you've been killing them up until now?" What about your reputation? What about lawsuits?

That's a tough one. I'd like to say, "Don't worry about it. Nothing bad will happen." I can't say that, even though, frankly, I think that. I actually haven't seen too many of the hospitals we work with hit such landmines when they start, openly, to work on these defects. But, the fact is that that reporter is exactly right. The harm is there. It has been there. The past deaths are real, not imagined. This is not a game.

The problem of admitting that we do harm goes to the core of our mission, our values, and, I guess, our courage. It is a bridge we have to cross, and we have to help sixteen hundred hospitals across it, too. In the IHI's IMPACT network, we now have dozens of hospitals already en route to life-saving changes. Indeed, their work is one of the foundations of my confidence that we can fly. Let me mention one pioneer, for example, one entire hospital system—the Ascension system—the largest Catholic hospital system in America, with sixty-seven hospitals. Last year, Ascension adopted three, consolidating corporate aims. They call them "Health Care That Is Safe," "Health Care That Works," and "Health Care That Leaves No One Behind."

Ascension says they want to have "no needless deaths." Do they really mean it? Yes, they mean it. I attended a meeting at which Ascension's CEO, Tony Tersigni, told five hundred of his managers, executives, and board members that needless deaths do occur at an unacceptable rate in Ascension, and that their strategy includes stopping them measurably and by a deadline. He didn't mean that Ascension was any worse than the rest of American health care; he was just telling the truth. If he can do it, so can you. We invited Ascension to bring a special display of their work here, and you can visit it this week. I hope you will.

We're going to have to say, "Come to the edge." And lots are going to say, "We are afraid." And still, we'll say, "Come to the edge." And we'll push them. And, like Ascension, they'll fly.

Wrong Thing Number Five: The doctors will never buy this. Sure, I am going to ask our medical staff to standardize their practice, to give up some of their autonomy, to pursue a psychotic goal the first step toward which is to admit openly that people die needlessly now. No way. The needless death I'm trying to avoid is my own.

Think again. Why is it that so many doctors and nurses seem so increasingly disaffected, so demoralized even though they are pursuing the life's work they chose? Why has money become the driving issue, and conflict the driving pattern?

I think that joy in work requires meaning in work. When the meaning dissolves, the joy evaporates. Let's save one hundred thousand lives. Let's do that together. Let's roll up our sleeves to fight disease, not each other. I do think the doctors will buy this. So will the nurses. In fact, they are waiting for this. I think this is the meaning in work that, unspoken, can get displaced by lower needs. I don't feel naïve about this; I don't think everybody will join. But some will; many will. If one doctor in five, one nurse in five, said, "Yes, that sounds worth my time—I'll take my share of the load—how can I help—what do you need me to do?"—that will be enough, plenty enough.

Wrong Thing Six is a tough one: What about you? This Campaign is about hospitals, and deaths that occur in only one sector of our health care system. What if you work in an office practice, or mental health, or nursing homes, or rehabilitation, or preventive medicine? How can you play if you are from another country?

Let me take a minute and speak first directly to the doctors—those of you out there right now who do want to help, but who don't happen to spend much time in hospitals. You are in office practices, maybe small ones. You'd like to help in the 100,000 Lives Campaign. But how?

You can be absolutely pivotal in this—whether you are hospital based, or not. Here are five things you can do starting right away that will give this Campaign legs and momentum.

First, if you are on a hospital medical staff, bring this Campaign to the attention of the staff, the medical director, the head of nursing, and the chief executive. Teach yourself the details and explain them to these people whenever and wherever you can. Be our agent—our precinct captain—for that hospital.

Second, do the same for the board of trustees of the hospital. Few board members know what is possible to achieve in improvement. A lot of them will believe it when they hear it from a physician in the community. Activating boards may be one of the best ways to start the ball rolling toward hospital-by-hospital change.

Third, when the time is right, invite the doctors in your community to work toward agreed standards of care—protocols for care—for conditions, like AMI and prevention of sepsis, where the results of doing that are life saving and known.

Fourth, ask your hospital to institute medication reconciliation procedures now for patients who are admitted to or discharged from the hospital.

Fifth, study and change your own practice. In your office setting, try to work on reliable composites, not just components. Use protocols to guide your own care toward high reliability. I think you will soon find yourself acting as a mentor to many of your peers.

I don't have an easy answer for everyone outside hospitals who might want to help the Campaign. We do have to start somewhere, and hospitals do have the biggest hazards. They need to build the highest dikes. It's a good place to start. But, let me share a secret. All the "No needless" aims count, every one of them. Deaths count, but so does pain, and delay, and helplessness, and waste, and inequity. And, if you promise to keep it a secret, I will tell you that this 100,000 Lives Campaign is only a start. This isn't an event; it's a movement. This is only the first of our candidates. We've got a whole slate ahead: reducing pain, helping in end-of-life care, involving patients in shared decisions, reducing waits and delays, tackling excess cost and waste, closing racial and ethnic gaps in health. And other countries will become involved. I would love to see Campaigns get started in Canada, the UK, and elsewhere.

Wrong Thing Seven may be this: What if we fail? What if we go out there promising one hundred thousand lives saved—sixteen hundred hospitals on board—and we fall flat? What if we save only twenty thousand lives, or ten thousand, or maybe only five thousand? Or even fewer? Won't we look foolish?

Foolish? No. Failure? There is no failure. If we hit one hundred thousand, we will surely have the biggest celebration health care has seen in a long time, I promise you. And, you know what, if it's twenty thousand, we'll celebrate, anyway. In fact, champagne for ten thousand. How's that for failure?

We are not going to do this alone. We couldn't. The IHI alone surely isn't big enough. Luckily, many of the most important stakeholders in American health care share our sense of both urgency and possibility. In fact, we've been talking with lots of them for many months, making plans jointly with them. A lot of what can—and will—happen in this Campaign will happen through their efforts and vision, not ours, and I have asked a few of them to join me on stage today. They are—every one of them—extremely busy people, and the mere fact that they have been ready, willing, and able to show up here today is maybe the strongest testimony to what we can get done together.

Our guests are Dr. John C. Nelson, president of the American Medical Association, Bill Atkinson, chairman of the North Carolina Hospital Association, Barbara Blakeney, president of the American Nurses Association—the ANA, Sister Mary Jean Ryan, president and CEO of SSM Health Care, Dr. David Pryor, senior VP of the Ascension Health system, Dr. Jonathan Perlin, who heads the Veterans Healthcare Administration, Dr. Steve Jencks, who heads the quality functions for the Centers for Medicare & Medicaid Services—CMS, Dr. Dennis O'Leary, president of the Joint Commission on Accreditation of Healthcare Organizations, and Sorrel King of the Josie King Foundation.

I should mention as they join me here that we could literally have filled the stage with other leaders—organizations, heath care systems, and others—who have expressed interest in, and, in fact, have already begun, the changes that this Campaign will focus on. Not the least of these are the 176 members of IHI's IMPACT network, which I call our "Association for Change," who have been working at many of these changes for over a year now. Colleagues, thank you for taking the time to be here.

So, what happens next? Well, we're pretty confident many of you would like a chance to digest and talk about the Campaign with our partners here, faculty, your colleagues, and IHI Campaign staff. You can do so this evening. We'll answer questions and provide you with any additional information you need.

Also—this is very important—please look inside the Campaign packet for a form we need you to fill out. We'll use this to learn about your interest in the Campaign, and to contact you with more detailed information about officially enrolling.

Satellite participants: we invite you to go to our website for the same materials we've handed out here in Orlando, and you'll also find information about how to sign up.

In January, we're going to hold two informational phone calls about the Campaign. Details are again on the website and in your Campaign packets.

So, here is what we will do:

Starting today—starting here—we will begin to enroll what will become sixteen hundred American hospitals in a Campaign to save one hundred thousand lives by June 14, 2006. Each enrolled hospital will commit to adopting whatever of these six changes it can commit to—I hope most will choose all six; and we will welcome any hospital to contribute ideas for other changes to add to the common store of knowledge. When we hit a good one not on the original list of six, we will make it known to all. We—the IHI—in full partnership with the nation's Quality Improvement Organizations, CMS, and the Joint Commission—will offer help and guidance to any enrolled hospital that wants to study the "how" of those life-saving changes. That help will range from absolutely free information and interactive supports on our websites, to more intensive Collaboratives and participatory projects involving fees and tuitions to cover their costs, and to subsidize and support outreach to safety net and rural facilities unable to cover their own costs.

We will collect quantitative reports whenever possible from enrolled hospitals, keeping a tote board of results, publicly assessing and reporting on the accumulating benefit of changes in lives saved—both measured and estimated from process–outcome relationship models.

We will welcome all partners in this to take the burden of portions of the "field" work to reach sixteen hundred hospitals—systems like Ascension, SSM, Premier, VHA, HCA, and Tenet, associations like the Vermont and North Carolina Hospital Associations, and others who will act as state, ward, and precinct captains do in political campaigns—covering the action for their designated segments of the sixteen hundred.

And, we will celebrate. Starting with pizza, and ending with champagne. We will celebrate the importance of what we have undertaken to do, the courage of honesty, the joy of companionship, the cleverness of a field operation, and the results we will achieve. We will celebrate ourselves, because the patients whose lives we save cannot join us, because their names can never be known. Our contribution will be what did not happen to them. And, though they are unknown, we will know that mothers and fathers are at graduations and weddings they would have missed, and that grandchildren will know grandparents they might never have known, and holidays will be taken, and work completed, and books read, and symphonies heard, and gardens tended that, without our work, would have been only beds of weeds.

On the beautiful campus of Wellesley College in Massachusetts is a sundial that has this poem inscribed:

> The shadow by my finger cast,
> Divides the future from the past
> Behind its unreturning line,
> The vanished hour, no longer thine.
> Before it lies the unknown hour
> In darkness and beyond thine power.
> One hour alone is in thine hands,
> The now on which the shadow stands.
> One hour alone is in thine hands . . . the now.

Let's get started. Some is not a number, soon is not a time. One hundred thousand lives. Now.

FURTHER READING

Bellomo R, Goldsmith D, Uchino S, et al. A prospective before-and-after trial of a medical emergency team. *Med J Aust*. 2003 Sep 15;179(6):283–287.

Chapter 3

POWER

COMMENTARY

Dale Ann Micalizzi

WHEN DON BERWICK invited me to write a commentary
about this speech, his request brought tears to my eyes. I still
remember the day, shortly before the 2005 Forum, when Don
sent his speech to me to review. He had to convince me to go
public and allow him to tell my son Justin's story.

At the Forum, I sat in the front row, listening to Don
speak. Dr. Mark Rosenberg sat on one side of me and Sorrel
King on the other, and I held on to each of their legs for
support. I wouldn't let Sorrel get up when Don asked the
audience to stand in a moment of silence and apology for me,
because I wanted that moment of silence to be for Sorrel,
too—for her daughter Josie—for all children and families that
have been harmed by the medical care they received. I will
never forget that feeling of support as six thousand health
caregivers at the Forum stood in silence.

Later that morning, when I was a presenter at a Forum
session with Mark, Sorrel, and Linda Kenney for the first time
ever—except to preschoolers—the audience cried again.
Several local health caregivers attending that session
connected with me later; those from a Vermont hospital
partnered on projects with me immediately. They wanted me
to be part of the cure. Some physicians still remind me of that
special day when Don had the audience rise in unison for
families who had been harmed by their profession. Justin was

proud of his mom that day. I'm glad Don convinced me to
show up and bring all of myself.

As I was returning to my room alone later that day, a doc
walked out of one of the hotel restaurant bars and looked at
me and said angrily, "We don't want you here!," and walked
away. I didn't respond to his comment, but it has really never
left me. Despite all of the many wonderful comments I've
since received from doctors at my presentations, that
comment still lingers. I try and brush it off, but I always think
when I'm finished presenting that there is at least one
physician or nurse in the audience who doesn't want to hear
my shaky voice talk about what went wrong.

Back home after the Forum, leaders showed the video of
Don's "Power" keynote address at a health care conference
attended by the hospitals involved in Justin's care. The
moderator introduced me and asked me to stand; you could
hear a pin drop. I don't think such an encounter had ever
happened before. A nurse slipped me a card with her phone
number, saying she wanted to meet me in private, because she
would be "blacklisted" if her nurse leader saw her talking
with me. We met in a local café soon after, and I learned
some of the struggles that nurses face.

Things have not really changed much locally; no one
involved has ever come clean about what really happened
behind the closed doors of the OR when Justin arrested. Still
silence. Still waiting . . .

Being a patient safety advocate has not been an easy ride,
but I plug along and try to keep my eye on the ball of saving
other families from harm. The Paediatric International Patient
Safety and Quality Collaborative (PIPSQC) recently "crowned
me" their Pediatric Patient Safety Ambassador. We are
forming a group of professional advocates and families who
want to partner with hospitals to save children's lives. I don't
know how to be an ambassador, but like Don not knowing
how to be a knight, perhaps I can make a difference, too.

I just listened to the first-grade teacher from Newtown,
Connecticut [site of a mass shooting on December 14, 2012],
being interviewed about her class and learning from the
event . . . and becoming stronger because of it. Even though
I could see the hurt in her eyes, she was teaching the children

a lesson on being resilient and reminding them to focus on the kindness of others and giving back. That's what I try to do: focus on the power of kindness and how we can feel free to help each other and not be afraid to do what's right even when it's hard . . . really hard.

Our yearly IHI Forum Scholarships in Justin's memory have instilled in our beneficiaries the will to focus on patient safety and quality and to listen to patient/family stories and learn from them. I couldn't have done any of this work without Don Berwick, my Knight of Quality and Safety, who truly cares . . . even for a grieving stranger looking for answers when he knew that she might never receive them.

POWER

PLENARY ADDRESS
INSTITUTE FOR HEALTHCARE IMPROVEMENT
17TH ANNUAL NATIONAL FORUM ON QUALITY
IMPROVEMENT IN HEALTH CARE
ORLANDO, FLORIDA, DECEMBER 13, 2005

ONE DAY THIS June I was quietly minding my own business, when I got a phone call. A man said, "This is John Rankin, the British consul general in Boston. May I ask you a question?" Here was his question: "If Queen Elizabeth were to offer you an honorary knighthood, would you accept it?" I said, "Who is this? No, really . . . who is this? Is this Bob?" (He's my brother.) "Is this Ken?" (He's my weirdo best friend.) But it wasn't. It *was* Mr. John Rankin, the British consul general.

That was a really tough question. It's not an everyday question. If the queen of England offered to make me a knight, would I accept? Hmm . . . So I thought about it, and then I said, "Sure." I mean, why not? So, on December fifth—last week—at the British Embassy in Washington, D.C., the British ambassador Sir David Manning held an investiture ceremony certifying me as an Honorary Knight Commander of the British Empire.

It's a little tough. I'm walking down the corridors and I say, "Hello, how are you?," and they say, "Fine, how are you?" I say, "Fine, I'm a knight," and the conversation stops dead.

I looked up being a knight on Google. I found three things. The first thing you need to know is that a non-British subject who is honorarily knighted isn't allowed to use the title, "Sir." I'll be automatically "Sir Donald" if I become a British citizen, but, until then, it's still just plain, "Don." My wife would have been Lady Berwick, but she isn't. This doesn't seem to bother her very much—go figure.

Second, notwithstanding the "Sir" thing, I do have lots of privileges. For example, if you, or if most of you, are convicted of a capital crime in the UK, you will have no choice but to be hanged. Not I. As a knight, I can choose hanging *or* beheading. I find that a relief.

Third—this didn't actually come from Google, but from talking in London this summer with a few other knights—actually, several Sirs and a Dame—as we ate together at—yes—a round table. They tell me that British Airways tends to treat knights pretty well. All the other knights told me to make absolutely sure that British Airways knows about this.

I happened to be passing through Heathrow Airport on the way home. So, I went up to a friendly looking ticketing agent, and I said, "Excuse me. This is probably a bit irregular, but I thought maybe British Airways might want to know that Queen Elizabeth just made me a knight."

The agent smiled at me, and she asked, "Oh, really, that's nice. What for?"

I swallowed hard and said, "Well . . . for upgrades."

"No," she asked, "I mean for what were you made a knight?"

"Oh," I said, "for helping to improve the English National Health Service."

The air chilled. The ticket agent glared at me. "Oh, really?" she said. "Improving the NHS, are you? Let me tell you about my Chlamydia."

I will spare you the details, but you should know that, when it comes to her Chlamydia, this person has serious doubts about NHS quality. "I guess you're not done with your improving yet, are you, Sir," she said. I thought maybe I should tell her not to call me "Sir," but then I thought maybe that wasn't such a good idea. It also didn't seem like such a good idea right then to help sort out her Chlamydia issues. I eased away, with my boarding pass—economy.

Actually, the knighthood means a lot to me personally. So many people—colleagues of the IHI—have been working in the UK for now nearly a decade to modernize the NHS. The NHS is an equitable and universal health care system, free at the point of care, and deeply committed to primary care. I think the NHS is one of the great human health care endeavors on Earth. It can be an example for the whole world—an example, I must say, that the United States needs now more than most other countries do. Helping the NHS realize its full potential is a massive task, with lots of ups and downs, but it's been a thrill to have the chance to work with so many committed, gifted, and open-minded NHS leaders. I'm thinking of friends like Helen Bevan, John Oldham, Nigel Crisp, Alan Langlands, Liam Donaldson, David Fillingham, Carol Black, and many,

many more. The actual truth is that, when Mr. Rankin called me, I was so moved that I cried.

But it started me thinking. Thinking about power. The nature of power. After all—"Knight Commander"—what does that mean?

Well, first, as much as my narcissism may wish that it means something about my power—my control—forget about it. There are, I suppose, actual halls of power in our nation—halls of great wealth, great armies, great political leverage. I'm not there. I assure you, I am *not* there.

But, our shared mission—to improve health care, all over the world—is a gigantic one, and it absolutely does need power. Lo and behold, we can see power. Look at the 100,000 Lives Campaign that IHI launched almost exactly one year ago, right here in Orlando, at last year's National Forum. It was only an idea—an uncertain, provocative idea. We went way out on a limb. The IHI had survived our first fourteen years of life, and we decided—what the heck—maybe it was time to try to start a wildfire blazing toward results at a full, national scale.

Starting small *would* have been much more prudent. But, we decided to pour gas on the flames. We said we would reduce needless deaths. We said one hundred thousand people would leave the hospital every year who otherwise would have died. We set a deadline—June 14, 2006—arbitrarily, because we thought a deadline was necessary. And we based the scientific platform for that goal on six changes in hospital care, each with a proven track record: Rapid Response Teams, reliable care for heart attacks, medication reconciliation procedures, and bundles of reliable care to prevent—maybe even eliminate—three types of killer infections: surgical site infections, ventilator-associated pneumonias, and central intravenous line bacteremia. We said that those changes could get us to that goal—one hundred thousand—if (and this was the big risk) something like sixteen hundred to two thousand hospitals signed on to do it.

Believe me, I lost sleep over this—ask Lady Berwick. The reasons it wouldn't work swamped the reasons it would. Hospital leaders would be afraid to admit publicly that needless deaths occur now. Doctors would fight standardization—cookbook medicine. The science would crumble under the spotlight. Patients who didn't die of our mistakes would die, anyway, of their diseases. Measurement, with proper case-mix adjustment, would prove technically impossible, even if hospitals would submit their mortality data to IHI, which they'd be too afraid to do, anyway. Competing demands from payers and regulators and so on would force this Campaign to the background—in fact, right off the table. And, most of all, there is no way we'd save these lives without levels of partnership and cooperation that would be out of reach in an industry that is plagued by anxiety, production pressures, lawsuits, rivalries.

We were wrong to worry. We were wildly wrong. We underestimated our colleagues. We underestimated *you*. We underestimated the good hearts, deep commitment, frustrated longings in American health care, the search for clarity, the pining for optimism, the recollection of why we work here, the intelligence, the good, good hearts. We underestimated the power. Not our power. Your power. We rubbed a lamp, and a genie popped out.

Bill Clinton said, "There is nothing wrong with America that what is right with America cannot fix." Well, I'll tell you, I am now absolutely convinced that "there is nothing wrong with American health care that what's right with American health care cannot fix." You're proving it—or you *can* prove it.

Two thousand, nine hundred, and eighty-nine hospitals signed up for the 100,000 Lives Campaign. They took the first step: enrollment—the pledge to change their care to save lives. Their pledge is public—their names are on IHI's website—and it came from the top—it's a pledge from senior leaders.

The second step—after enrollment—is harder, and not everybody has made it yet. It's to count—to count out loud. To count deaths. To count the rate of mortality, and to report it to us at IHI. Stare the number in the face in your organizations like an enemy across a battlefield—with steely gaze and firm purpose. Like Knight Commanders of the British Empire do. Like Aragorn does when he is fighting the Orcs. So far, of the 2,989 hospitals in the Campaign, 74 percent have reported their mortality data to us. That's a stunning start in a very, very nervous industry.

The third step is where the lives actually get saved—by actually changing care—"execution." We need serious, wise adaptation of every change to every local context. We've learned a ton about such local execution. Our Campaign field staff have been crisscrossing the United States for months, visiting hospitals and the coalitions—the "Nodes"—that are helping us reach the hospitals. What we've been finding is something is bigger and better than I've ever seen before in my career in health care.

Listen to a few stories from the field in the 100,000 Lives Campaign:

- In Madison, Wisconsin, the state Node leaders took the IHI Campaign team to the University of Wisconsin stadium. There, they had outlined in yellow balloons six thousand seats. That's the number of lives that they intend to save in Wisconsin this year and every year.

- In Kansas City, Kansas, our team met Jennifer McClanahan. A Rapid Response Team at Kansas University Medical Center saved her life—at least she and they think so. A transport technician alerted the team.

- Parkview Hospital, in Fort Wayne, Indiana, sent me their customized "100,000 Lives" Campaign button. They are sort of marrying their home to our home, and they're committing to change.

Where did this come from? Where did this genie come from? Where did all this power come from?

At last year's Forum, just as we were announcing the Campaign, Rose Lindsey [cochair of IHI's 2004 National Forum] announced that a wonderful thing had happened for my daughter Jessica and our family: Jessica was admitted to medical school.

She started this September, and she told me a story about her first week that I want to share with you.

Jessica is studying anatomy. Anatomy in medical school isn't just a topic; it's a rite of passage. It's where most future doctors face death up-close for the first time—in the lab where they meet their "donor" cadaver. Dissecting a human body will imprint memories on their minds that they're going to rely on as they deal with living bodies for the rest of their careers. You know where the subclavian vein is, you know how the pleura attach to the lung, how the mitral valve is tethered to the endocardium, how far back in the peritoneum the kidneys lie—because this once—maybe only this once—you actually saw it.

The donors—the people who give their bodies—decided to help a future that they'll never see. Yale School of Medicine, where Jessica is learning now, helps the students to acknowledge their gift, beginning when anatomy class starts, and ending in a ceremony of thankfulness to the donors at the end of the year.

Anatomy lab is a shocker. It would be for anyone, but imagine what it's like for a twenty-three-year-old kid. It totally reframes your relationship to death, to the body. Yale tries to help the students to accept—to value—their feelings, not deny them—to bring their whole selves to their work. It used to be taught—I was taught—that professionalism required distance. That the doctor shouldn't let herself feel too close to her patient, or else she'll become the victim of her feelings, and lose objectivity.

That wasn't smart. Why would we ever teach that these deep emotions, awakened in young people who are committing themselves to the relief of suffering, need to be pushed aside, or even that they *can* be pushed aside? We know better now—Yale knows better now. (I think that maybe the nursing profession, actually, has known it a lot longer.) And so the message Jessica is getting is much more affirming, much more integrating. It'll make her a better doctor. The message is, "Show up." "Bring all of you here." The meeting of two human beings—two *complete* human beings—has a power to heal that distant, defended relationships cannot have. Never, never, never lose the technical edge; bring your skill and knowledge fully to the patient. Never, never, never let your asymmetrical power and your human fantasies carry you over the ethical line between you and the patient. But, also, never, never, never forget that you and your patients share in common souls, and spirits, and that, as they suffer, so do you suffer; as they fear, so do you fear, and as they hope, so do you hope. And, crucially, as they err, so do you err. Your white coat is a coat.

In Jessica's orientation, her anatomy professor, Larry Rizzolo, told about a student a few years ago who, facing her donor cadaver for the first time, felt nothing. That went on for weeks. She didn't feel fear, or sadness, or confusion, like many of her classmates were feeling. Not, that is, until the day she finished the dissection from the front of the body. Then, she turned her donor over, and there she saw it, on the donor's back: a Band-Aid.

And *then* she cried. The Band-Aid did it. It had the power to unleash the tears. Objects—things—don't need Band-Aids. *People* do. Her donor had lived.

A big, harsh wave is sweeping over health care today: rapid movement toward market forces and more competition, pay for performance, public reporting of quality, and making consumers cost sensitive. There's a reason. It's because, despite its biotechnical glory, health care isn't meeting social needs. Ford and GM are both at the brink of corporate disaster, and a lot of the reason is that health care and retiree benefit costs, waste and defects in health care have driven them there. In its United States market, Starbucks spends more on health care than on coffee products. My good friend Dennis O'Leary, the president of the Joint Commission and one of the most clear-headed leaders in American health care today, says that the best advice he has for an American patient to protect his or her safety in the hospital is to bring a loved one with them as a guard. Bring a guard to our place of healing! And I agree with Dennis.

The harsh wave of policy change is entirely understandable. Doesn't a system out of control need controls put on it? Doesn't a system that's not accountable for defects need to be made accountable? Shouldn't people and organizations with opaque performance be made transparent, forced into glaring daylight so that everybody can see the truth about the care?

Public reporting, quality measurement, balanced scorecards, market forces, pay for performance, even consumer choice—these are the harvest in policy of frustration with a care system in the United States that is taking an unfair share of social resources for an uncertain and unproven benefit, a system that often harms the people it should serve. And, it's not just in the United States. The same list of policies is now appearing in local idioms all over the world.

This is a search for power. These policies come from a conventional wisdom, which says that we can tame this wild beast with the right bridles of accountability, market force, and transparency.

Is that going to work? I don't know. Maybe it'll help. I have no doubt at all that the new policy era will achieve a new level of compliance. But, will it achieve a new level of healing? Will it give us a new system of care? The one we need? Is it powerful enough for that amount of change?

I don't think so. I think it's an incomplete plan. I don't think it has the power. Not because it will fail to accomplish a great deal, but because it will fail to accomplish the most important deal. If we aren't careful, in fact, I think that this regime of accountability, markets, pay for performance, and public reports could take the stuffing right out of us; it could unplug the power we need to do this job of healing right. Band-Aid power.

Where could the power lie? The answer is not at all comfortable. It isn't easy. In fact, markets would be a ton easier.

I think maybe Justin Micalizzi has the power. He was eleven years old when he died. His mother, Dale, sent me an email two years ago. This is part of it:

> On January 15, 2001, Justin, a healthy 11-year-old boy, was taken into surgery to incise and drain a swollen ankle. He was dead by 7:55 a.m. the next morning, leaving behind two grieving and bewildered parents who desperately wanted to know why their son had died. But medical care was to fail them twice—first their son died, and then no one would explain to them why.
>
> I know the chaos, the nursing shortages, overtime, the financial obligations, the insurance company guidelines, and the arrogance that

interferes with the quality of care. I have worked in health care and education for over 20 years. I also know, when it came time for my son's surgery, you remove the chaos. You develop a team effort to review all information and establish a plan. You openly communicate between specialists, remove arrogance and intimidation, and have a common goal to heal. It is your obligation to complete checklists, check and double check medications and dosages, assign a nursing team, and treat every case as a possible emergency with the patient as your ONLY focus. Look at the child; listen to the parents; and use common sense and professional judgment when making all decisions. Slow down! You are holding my child's life in your hands. Justin WAS important and should have been important to his health care providers also. I trusted you.

The hospital failed us, the nurses who were his advocates failed us, and the technicians . . . failed us. . . . [T]he surgeon . . . failed us. The health department failed us. . . . The hospital CEO failed us. . . . Error upon accepted error killed my son and my faith in a medical system that was meant to comfort and heal. We will not let this happen to another family. The pain is unbearable.

There are tears in your eyes, as there are tears in mine. There have been every time I have reread this—a hundred times—since the moment Mrs. Micalizzi sent it to me. She is not alone. Mrs. Micalizzi stands with thousands—tens of thousands—of patients and loved ones who are asking us why this has happened. How could this happen?

This isn't a simple matter. If Justin's death could be traced to a single, identifiable cause—an obvious error—a mislabeled drug—if we knew for sure how he died, somehow this story would be much simpler. We could blame a person or a process, declare the defect unacceptable, and manage it away, sad that Justin paid the price of our inattention. But, this story doesn't let us off the hook so easily. That's because we don't know why Justin died. The hospital says—and I believe them—that they have turned over every rock looking for a culprit error, and they can't find one. An eleven-year-old boy came to them alive and thriving (Justin's mother says he was "charismatic"), and he died in their hands. And they don't know why. For me, the hardest thing I need to tell his mother is that I think we will never know.

What is their duty? What is our duty? It is double.

Here is our first duty: Take responsibility for what happens on our watch, despite our ignorance and even when our search for a cause is unfruitful. Our duty is never, ever, ever to be willing to sleep soundly on the theory that "bad things happen." It is to convert every tragedy we can into a needless one—to create the possibility of repair and prevention where none at first exists. I do not accept the classification of harm to our patients as "preventable" or "unpreventable." The enemy is not error; it is injury. We will mature in our mission to improve safety if and when we accept the responsibility to *make* harm preventable. That job comes with the territory of leadership. Those who can't accept it should not lightly choose to lead. I once phoned the head of safety for Boston's enormous public works project—the "Big Dig"—to ask him how they were approaching worker safety. Here is what he told me: "The first rule of safety is 'zero,'" he said. "When you accept any injury as inevitable, you are on the road to failure."

The first job is to accept responsibility for Justin's death, even when we cannot yet know why it happened. We don't know why he died. But, that's exactly why I want to think with you about Justin. I do not think that it is our job to explain that Justin had to die; it is to accept responsibility because we did not save him.

Our second duty, as always, is to heal as best we can. Justin's death left two communities deeply wounded—his family and the workforce that tried to help him. Always heal. Healing depends on honest, open disclosure, conversation, shared tears, and offers and promises to do absolutely everything in our human power to protect those who will follow Justin into our risk-filled care. Like Jessica is being taught, we need to show up—bring all of ourselves. Healing can't occur in a context of denial, mutual recrimination, silence, or self-defense. It can't occur without deep introspection, apology, shared grief, and, eventually, somehow, trust.

This means not just—or even *mainly*—that injured patients and families should learn again to trust their caregivers. Sometimes that's impossible. It is much more crucial that the caregivers and the leaders of their organizations learn to trust in the intelligence, generosity, and creative capacity of the very people whom they have injured. It means inviting into the hearts of our organizations and the presence of our healers the patients and families whose stories, ideas, observations, and vision can help to guide us into new and better work. I don't know if Justin's mother can ever forgive us for what we cannot explain; she has no duty to do that. But, I do know this; she is with us this morning. Despite her pain, she wants to help. Mrs. Micalizzi has asked me to read aloud the names of other children who have been injured in health care, and whose parents have networked their way to her for mutual support.

They are Monica, Charlotte, Jessica, Jennifer, Seth, Josie, Claire, Erin, Stephanie, Lewis, Lisa, Katie, Libby, and Michael.

Let me tell you something very important. Of all of the lessons from the 100,000 Lives Campaign, this could be the most important one. As hospital after hospital has signed on, pledged to reduce needless deaths, and, 71 percent of the time, reported its death rates, we have not yet seen in the press or public testimony a *single* case of recrimination, startled outrage, or even severe impatience. This is a fundamental finding from the Campaign. The public is *not* becoming outraged when we get honest. The public—even the press—has cut us slack, plenty enough slack, to get about this job, and even, incredibly, generously, graciously, they have so far given us a "high sign." They're encouraging the work that they would have every right to expect we had begun decades and decades ago. Like Mrs. Micalizzi, they want us to succeed, in part to show the only real respect we can for their irrecoverable loss.

We need to return the favor by accepting the duty. May I please ask you to stand here, right now, for a moment of silence, to reflect on the loss of Justin, and to share with Mrs. Micalizzi the grief and regret that this should have happened?

Some of you stood in regret; others, even, in apology. I apologize. I so wish I could apologize to Justin, himself, but that chance is lost. We *can* apologize to Mrs. Micalizzi. We *can* say we are sorry. It happened on our watch. No one in this room, I suspect, actually took care of Justin directly, but I believe that we can and should accept collective responsibility for not yet having built a health care world safe enough for him, and for tens of thousands of patients and families who are injured in our care. Mrs. Micalizzi, I am so, so sorry.

This is power. Band-Aid power. Feel what happens—feel what we intend—feel what we can try—not because of a number, or pay for performance, or a report card, or a market. This is power of a totally different, far, far better sort. It will lead us to do not what we must, but what we should.

Now, we can start. For, after the regret, after the tears, comes the possibility. It is not enough—it will not change anything—merely to see Justin's face. Now, we need the power of hope.

Hope is power. Optimism—joined with regret—not regret alone, starts change.

The best recipe for power that I have encountered I heard first from Tom Nolan, my chief guide in the improvement jungle. If you have been to an IHI meeting in the past few years, you probably have already heard it: "Will, ideas, and execution." That's what it takes to change a large system—what it will take to change health care. The will comes both from our hearts and from our fears. It comes from seeing the Band-Aid, from mourning Justin. It is essential.

But will lies fallow, frustrated, without ideas. The other way—the new way—is about what we *could* do when we combine will with ideas. Luckily, we have among us both scientists and optimists—knowledge pioneers and action pioneers.

If you haven't met Lee Vanderpool [senior director, IT, at Dominican Hospital], you really should. He sent me an email this month:

> Dear Friends at IHI—
>
> On October 12, 2005, the team of caregivers at Dominican Hospital reached a key milestone of zero cases of ventilator-associated pneumonia for one year. In our weekly critical care team meeting, we acknowledged our roots in the IHI Critical Care Collaborative, and the lofty goals that we set with you in 2002. You may remember our earlier goal of setting a 100-day VAP-free road trip that ended at day 93 with a very compromised botulism patient, so this week's result has been particularly rewarding. We remain guardedly optimistic that our processes are sound, and our goal is to hold the gains. Indeed, we have had four cases of VAP over the past 27 months.

See the words. "Lofty goals." "Particularly rewarding." "Guardedly optimistic." These aren't accidental expressions. They are driven—hopeful. They raise this question: "If they can, why can't you?"

If you haven't met Sherry Tishenor, from St. Joseph Hospital, in Lexington, Kentucky, you really should. I first met her only a couple of months ago. That's because her hospital, a member of IHI's IMPACT network, has had one of the fastest and largest reductions in standardized mortality rate that we have recently seen—a decline of thirty-one points on a scale where the American average standardized hospital death rate is one hundred. Thirty-one points! I wanted to know how they did that. So, I asked.

Sherry left me speechless. They have simply pulled out all the stops—every Campaign intervention, innovations on hazardous medications, relentless pursuit of every single adverse case until they understand deeply why. They do not regard needless death as inevitable. They regard needless death as a worthy and constant enemy, against which they will be samurai. Sherry uses an expression that captivated me: "Things that get you dead . . ." She hates those things, and she enlists everybody around her to wage war on those things. Heparin can get you dead, and so St. Joseph now treats heparin just like it treats a chemotherapy agent. A 31 percent decline in mortality! Let me ask you: If Sherry can, why can't we?

If you haven't met the people of Harborview Medical Center in Seattle, you really should. There, they have implemented Rapid Response Teams in the fastest rollout I've seen yet. In their first two weeks, they achieved fifty-five Rapid Response Team calls—that is over twice as many per thousand admissions as the best prior rate I knew. Our Australian colleagues say that their best sites call Medical Emergency Teams at the rate of about twenty-five times per thousand admissions. Harborview doubled that in their first two weeks. If they can, why can't we all?

With thousands working at change, I can't possibly tip my hat to each individually, but I just can't resist extending the list a bit.

- Fairview Southdale in Edina, Minnesota, treats over seven hundred heart attack patients a year. The CMS goal for door-to-balloon time for coronary stents is 120 minutes. The AHA/ACC goal is 90 minutes. Fairview Southdale's average is 70 minutes.

- Advocate Good Samaritan Hospital outside Chicago averages 59 minutes.

- Swedish Medical Center in Seattle has six ICUs in three campuses. They went 168 days without a ventilator-associated pneumonia, reduced overall VAP rates by 68 percent, and saved $720,000.

- The University of Rochester's Strong Memorial Hospital went 492 days in their cardiovascular ICU without a ventilator pneumonia.

- Our Lady of Lourdes Medical Center in Binghamton, New York, went 290 days without a VAP and 166 days without a central line infection.

- Indianapolis Heart Hospital, part of Bill Corley's Community Hospitals of Indiana, went twenty-five months without a central line infection, and they're still counting.

- Southwestern Vermont Medical Center—one full year without a central line infection.

- Denver Health Medical Center, providing 42 percent of the uncompensated care in their region—four months without a VAP.

- Overlake Hospital Medical Center in Bellevue, Washington— VAPs down by 90 percent, central line infections by 74 percent, an estimated forty-five patients with harm averted, and $2 million in savings.

- Virginia Mason Medical Center has had no preventable codes outside the ICU in five of the past seven months.

- Seton Medical Center in Austin, Texas, implemented Rapid Response Teams eighteen months ago. They have had only five codes outside their ICU between June and November.

- North Country Regional Hospital in North Central Minnesota, with 117 beds, started Rapid Response Teams in April and has had no codes outside the ICU since.

- Ridgeview Medical Center in Waconia, Minnesota, has really racked up the successes. Year to date in September, their composite compliance with the AMI care standards—100 percent; for heart failure—99 percent; for community-acquired pneumonia—97 percent. No central line infections in twenty-four months. No ventilator pneumonias in twenty-four months. Rapid response in place with no out-of-CCU codes since August. And a median door-to-balloon time of ninety-one minutes, which may not sound too impressive until you know that the cardiac catheterization facility they use is thirty-one miles away from the hospital.

- National ICU care leader Peter Pronovost reported recently on accumulated experience in preventing central line infections in seventy hospitals. The harvest: 1,578 lives saved; 81,020 hospital days and over $165 million in costs averted.

You stood a few moments ago in regret, with sorrow that you share for the loss of Justin. On the floor of Harborview Medical Center's main lobby are many quotations from cultures around the world. One says this: "Sorrow shared is halved; joy shared is doubled." You shared the sorrow. Share the joy. Can I invite you to stand again in hope? Thank Lee Vanderpool and Dominican. Thank Sherry Tishenor and St. Joseph Hospital. Thank Harborview. Thank Ridgeview. Honor what they give to us—the fresh start—the sense of possibility.

Why has the 100,000 Lives Campaign attracted 2,989 hospitals—samurai against things that get you dead? The answer is, first, regret, and, second, optimism. They don't just hate what has happened; they believe they can put an end to it. And all of this happens with not a nickel of pay for performance, not a jot of enforced accountability, not a byte of involuntary measurement. It is entirely, 100 percent, authentically, willed from within.

Will, ideas, and then execution. From facing our duty, from apology, comes will. From the examples of the pioneers comes the optimism of ideas. Now, if Tom Nolan is right, we are just one element away from success. That step is execution, the hardest step, commitment to day-to-day detail, the hard work of making the change. What good is a knight without a good fight?

The 100,000 Lives Campaign asks for execution on a scale we haven't ever previously imagined. We're asking, "If *there*, then why not *everywhere*?" This Campaign calls on thousands of places and tens of thousands of people to attend to details—to make change real.

This is the power of taking action. In a *New York Times* op-ed piece by Robert Kaplan, I read the following line, which Kaplan says is common among soldiers: "Amateurs discuss strategy; professionals discuss logistics."

Take a closer look at Harborview. Remember the Rapid Response Team roll-out there? Well, when our team visited, we found these pads on the med-surg units. Slips of yellow paper. One side lists the criteria for calling a Rapid Response Team, and a little coaching on the communications tool called SBAR—Situation-Background-Assessment-Recommendation. We stole SBAR from the military. It helps people at all levels talk to each other efficiently and boldly when clear communications matter most. Anyone at Harborview can use this form to call the team, and the back of the form is the feedback report on that call that goes into the quality improvement staff to keep tabs on the system and improve it.

You need to see a line—it goes from Justin's tragedy, to Australian researchers and our rapid response pioneers, to Harborview's actions, to this little slip of paper. It goes all the way from the need to the logistics—right down to the details. "Amateurs discuss strategy; professionals discuss logistics." What are the logistics—the deeds—the details of hard, specific work that are going to translate your optimism into daily work?

Let's not be naïve about this. Signing up for the Campaign is easy—just a piece of paper. Watching samurai from afar is easy, too. It's a spectator sport. But, saving one hundred thousand lives is just not delegable. It's a *contact* sport. In fact, some of my Campaign colleagues aren't buying the champagne just yet. Here is an email one sent me a few weeks ago:

> For lack of a better way to say it, there is a lot of fake will or symbolic
> will [among Campaign participants] . . . *insofar as execution is the*
> *ultimate measure of will.* . . . For all of the genuine commitment we've
> observed in the field, we've observed a lot of cynicism, too, when
> hospitals and systems actively advertise their involvement and then
> take no real action. People need to have that moment where they look
> in the mirror and ask themselves if they're serious about completely
> eradicating the processes that kill people now.

This is "that moment." Help me out here. I want to cure this guy's
skepticism, but that doesn't depend on me. It depends on all of us. It
depends on going beyond enrollment. Beyond ideas. "Insofar as execution is the ultimate measure of will . . ."

Let's take a closer look at the 100,000 Lives Campaign scorecard. We
have thrilling stories to tell by now—case by case—Harborview, Dominican, Ridgeview. But, what's the whole pattern so far? Here are the
numbers:

- We have 2,989 hospitals signed up for the Campaign.
- If we cross-walk that list to the American Hospital Association
  data set, those hospitals will account for about thirty million
  discharges this year—over 90 percent of all hospital discharges in
  America.
- To achieve one hundred thousand lives saved, those hospitals will
  have to reduce deaths by two per thousand discharges.
- Among hospitals reporting their plans for process changes, the
  distribution of participation in Campaign planks is this:
  - Rapid Response Teams: 59 percent
  - AMI care reliability: 77 percent
  - Medication reconciliation: 73 percent
  - Surgical site infection prevention: 72 percent
  - Ventilator Bundle: 67 percent
  - Central Line Bundle: 65 percent
- As of last count, 2,198 hospitals are sending IHI their mortality
  data—74 percent of those enrolled. Tracking the death rates only
  in the reporting hospitals, and adjusting for the rising case mix
  index through time, we now have reports of 14,679 deaths
  averted—in hand—in the first eight months of the Campaign. By
  the end of the first year, that means we should have 32,397 lives
  saved in the 2,989 hospitals.

- We can extrapolate that experience to the end of the Campaign using several different models. For example, if we assume that, between now and the end of the Campaign, all 2,989 hospitals will continue to save lives at the same rate as those that have already reported, then the Campaign members will reduce deaths by 48,581 by June 14, 2006. But, hospital performance seems to be improving steadily over time so far. If we assume that that improvement continues to accelerate through June 2006, extrapolated to all 2,989 hospitals, 98,094 lives will be saved.

Not bad. Not bad at all. Will, ideas, and the first wave of execution. But, let me be clear, that result is not yet in the bag . . . not at all. We didn't say 48,581. We said one hundred thousand. And 100,000 minus 48,581 leaves 51,419. Getting to one hundred thousand is going to involve a lot more work. I can't make you knights, but you are all knights in my eyes. And, when a knight *takes* a job, he *does* the job. Can you imagine Sir Francis Drake telling Queen Elizabeth that he made it to, say, Brazil, and felt that that was, Your Royal Highness, good enough? We don't do that.

Let's get it done. It can be done. It's will, ideas, execution. But, now, actually, it's all come down to one of those: execution.

Let's take execution seriously—all of us. I know that all of you in the Campaign really, really, really would love to announce at our International Hospital Summit in Atlanta, Georgia, on June 14, 2006, that we hit—beat—our target—all together—one hundred thousand lives. On our current path, we'll have gains, but we will fall short. Let's not. Do this, please. Make it real.

Five tasks, you samurai.

Task One: *Reaffirm* your commitment to the Campaign. If you're not engaged in all six key interventions now, expand to all six. Better still, this is the time to add in any other improvements you believe will help contribute to the goals of the Campaign. We are seeing innovators emerge to do just that in many locales. Blood sugar control looks promising; so does a renewed emphasis on reliable treatment of sepsis. We are, in fact, establishing a set of cutting-edge teams to study and report on enhancements to the six core interventions. Join one; or at least follow what happens closely.

If you are a board member or a hospital executive, when I talk about reaffirming your commitment to the Campaign, I'm looking, especially, at you. Create urgency. Expect your organization to be at the vanguard in securing the Campaign interventions and in getting the results.

Task Two: If you haven't done so yet, *assign responsibility*. Now is the time for your board and executives to assign a specific, senior person to lead your Campaign work between now and June. Create a captaincy, and give that leader resources and visibility to drive the needed process changes in the affected clinical units.

Task Three: *Report* your mortality data to IHI. We especially need your mortality data. But, we'd also love to get your process data if that's at all possible for you. Enrollment is fine, but it isn't enough. Counting what we accomplish isn't a frill; it's essential. So far, 26 percent of Campaign participants are still not sending their monthly mortality data in. Without it, how can we know if we are getting to our goal as a nation, and how can they know if they are getting to their goal as an organization? It's time to turn that corner. Please take this question seriously: If you aren't sending in your mortality data, are you really in the Campaign, or not? If you are sending the data, don't let up.

Task Four: *Review* your work. Review what you are doing in the Campaign locally, every day, with urgency. This is the time to integrate detailed Campaign progress reviews into the work of every single stakeholder in the hospital—boards, leaders, quality managers, front-line teams. I think the senior leaders of your organization should review your Campaign work weekly or even more often for the next six months, starting right now. Ask if your processes really are changing—really! Ask if you are seeing cycle-by-cycle improvements in implementation—really!

Task Five: *Join in* the learning processes of the Campaign broadly, thoroughly. We can connect you with your peer organizations in our new mentor network, and some of them may well be doing better at implementation than you are. They can guide and coach you, but only if you ask. Use the Campaign website, and mine it for all you can for examples of effective implementation. If you are stalled, get unstalled, by finding and using the lessons being learned by others in the United States. We are a large country, and somewhere someone has almost certainly solved whatever problem is holding you back.

Now, a lot of you don't work in hospitals. And, so let me also say a special word to the many of you here who don't. Time and again, even with the limited range of the Campaign interventions, the whole continuum of health care rides into view. You can't get heart attacks treated promptly if people out there in the community don't understand and respond to early warning signs. And, of course, we'd have a lot fewer heart attacks to treat if proper control of hypertension, cholesterol, and diabetes were reliable. Medication reconciliation is probably more important outside hospitals' walls than within them. And better infection control reaches far upstream right into habits of antibiotic overuse in the community at large. I invite—I urge—all the people in our continuum of care to take the Campaign thinking dead center, wherever you work. For the longer haul, I am increasingly excited by the thought that this Campaign can open the door to even more and wider Campaigns ahead, maybe very soon, other Campaigns that will grapple with issues in chronic disease care, social and ethnic disparities, and prevention, with just as much energy as this first Campaign is showing. To be really bold, maybe, just *maybe*, in this great wave of enrollment and rededication, we have for the first time the seeds of something we really need: an American health care system worthy of the name "system."

That's your assignment. Make the skeptics eat crow with their champagne. And remember, I'm a knight. I have a lance. Well, I couldn't get in on the airplane but I'm going to get a lance. Do it.

As for me, though I am a skeptic still, I find plenty of reason for hope. Let me close with a story that gives you a taste of what I can taste.

Recall the Campaign's transcontinental bus tour in October. We stopped in fifteen cities for meetings, rallies, and hospital visits. We stopped in Washington, and Chicago, in Topeka, and Boise, as many stops as we could squeeze in, and I wish we had had time for many, many more. And we ended in Seattle. Now, on the Campaign tour, our team had many inspiring moments, as hospital after hospital showed its work and lessons learned. I've got to tell you, Seattle looks special. It's inspiring, because almost every player in that city is breaking new ground in improvement: Virginia Mason, Harborview, Group Health Cooperative, Swedish, Overlake, the University Hospital, every single one.

Lots of those bus tour moments stand out for me, but there was one in particular that I know I'll never forget. It was in a large hall, with four hundred or so people there from hospitals all over Washington—our amazing Node there has enrolled every single one of the acute care hospitals in the state. I spoke, and then, in the question-and-answer period a man rose. "I am the CMO of a large hospital," he said, naming the hospital—which everybody in the room knew and many compete with. "We owe you 360 lives by June 14, 2006." That was the share he and his colleagues had computed would represent their proportional contribution to the one hundred thousand. "We owe you 360 lives, and that means that we need to hit a benchmark of 200 lives saved by December." So, they were managing their trajectory. Amazing. "But," he said, "so far, we've only got sixty-six. We're worried. We're off schedule. Do you really think we can do it?"

There was silence. I was thinking. I mean, after all, I don't know for sure if they can do it. *We* can do it—our *nation* can do it. But, can *he* do it? Can *that hospital* do it? Well, that depends on lots of things that I don't know—that I can't know: history, internal conflicts, local conditions, the will of their board, the distractions of their market, the busy-ness of everyday lives. Can they see the Band-Aid? What would they have done if Justin had died there? I was thinking, "What can I say that will both encourage him and show that I respect what he and his colleagues may have to grapple with?"

But, I never did answer. Because, in the silence, a person across the room spoke loudly from his seat, and everyone heard. "Sixty-six lives," the voice said. "Sixty-six lives. Thank you. Thank you so much." And the room filled with applause, an entire community of health care leaders, celebrating together, embracing one of their own—and the courage to try, the courage to count, the courage to be honest, and an achievement already worth a lifetime of effort.

And, I thought. How unafraid! How strong! How unstoppable! Now *that's* a knight! What power!

Chapter 4

MONT SAINTE-VICTOIRE

COMMENTARY

Jason Leitch, DDS, FDS, MPH

IN THE LAST few months of 2004, I stumbled across the Institute for Healthcare Improvement (IHI). I had never heard of IHI. I was trawling for funding to continue some research in my conventional clinical academic role in Glasgow, Scotland. I came across the Health Foundation and applied for their Quality Improvement Fellowship. I found myself, in the summer of 2005, with four other successful candidates beginning a one-year fellowship at IHI. That's when I first heard Don Berwick speak.

IHI fellows have the opportunity to attend the Harvard School of Public Health Summer Program and to participate in Maureen Bisognano's Quality Improvement course. Don was the guest speaker one Friday afternoon. I have a confession—I thought it was nonsense. Don talked of *Crossing the Quality Chasm*; Trigger Tools; harm rates that made my hair stand on end; deaths and adverse events "caused" by us—by the system I worked in and had been part of for fifteen years. I thought it was heresy!

In reality, Don was going easy on us that day. The challenge was even greater than he had expressed. He sent the IHI fellows out on the road to see the solutions. We travelled to Cincinnati Children's Hospital, Virginia Mason Medical

Center, Premier, and San Diego Children's Hospital. We saw reliable design, leadership, and person-centered care that made a real difference. We then returned home, after the IHI fellowship, to our health systems in the United Kingdom and the United States.

The fellows had been home for six months; attending the 2006 IHI National Forum was our first opportunity to reconnect in person with friends, IHI, and Don. We had been fellows at IHI during the 100,000 Lives Campaign and proud to be at the 2005 Forum to celebrate the Campaign's progress. But now we were back in our real jobs and it was hard. How could we take what we had learned and use it—really use it—at the appropriately named coal-face, at the front line of health care?

In retrospect, I can now see that the 5 Million Lives Campaign announced in Don's 2006 National Forum speech and its predecessor, the 100,000 Lives Campaign, have led to broader changes than those previously seen in the United States. The Campaigns have been a catalyst for global change in health care delivery. I have been privileged to be involved in a number of extensions of this work around the world.

Around the time of Don's 2006 speech, a group of leaders in Scotland had been considering how to make Scotland's hospital care safer. The Scottish Patient Safety Programme (SPSP) was launched in May 2007, five months after this speech. SPSP has now spread to all of Scotland's hospitals and to maternity care, mental health, and primary and community care.

Similar work is underway in Denmark, Wales, and Norway, just to name a few countries. The focus of these programs is, in large part, the Campaign "planks" Don introduced in his 2006 Forum keynote—pressure ulcers, infections, and so on.

All of this work can trace its way back to the evidence-based interventions of IHI's Campaigns. Of course, the work has been contextualized for each country and each system, but these programs have one thing in common. They are engaging. I think there is a lot of nonsense spoken about clinical engagement. My experience is that clinicians are engaged when the work is engaging.

There is a story in Don's speech about a nurse who tells Don of her joy from being involved in the Campaign. I have had this same experience. A nearly retired diabetes physician told me he stayed in his post because SPSP had given him hope, and it was the greatest initiative in which he had been involved in forty years. A senior pediatric surgeon, in tears, told me stories of harm he had caused; he was filled with joy about something as simple as the surgical safety checklist introduced to him through SPSP and the difference it was making in his practice.

The work of improving health care delivery is relentless. It is global and it requires design. In this speech, Don talks of Cézanne's motif of Mont Sainte-Victoire and suggests that risk is our motif in health care—always present, always ready to harm or kill. The call to action in this 2006 speech still stands today. It is a call to relentless reliability; to listen to patients and families. It is, in particular, a call for boards of directors to take responsibility, and to transform leadership at all levels in health care. It requires action, design, and courage. Don "paints us a picture" of all three in this speech.

MONT SAINTE-VICTOIRE

PLENARY ADDRESS
INSTITUTE FOR HEALTHCARE IMPROVEMENT
18TH ANNUAL NATIONAL FORUM ON QUALITY
IMPROVEMENT IN HEALTH CARE
ORLANDO, FLORIDA, DECEMBER 12, 2006

YOUR WORK—ALL of your work—this year has been awesome. IHI has never been busier. Our IMPACT network has grown; our website gets eight thousand hits a day; we have more and more R&D programs, like Transforming Care at the Bedside, innovation communities in flow and reliability and disparities and perinatal care; new programs in ambulatory care and office practices; and a fantastic project on new levels of patient empowerment called New Health Partnerships. We have more and more health professions education students among us, including the Minnesota Clarion case competition winners from Virginia Commonwealth University, and twenty-eight students attending the Forum on scholarships through our Health Professions Education Collaborative. Our courses for executives and patient safety officers and improvement advisors are full. Premier, a longstanding IHI partner, won the Baldrige Award; and our international friends continue to multiply in Europe, Australia, New Zealand, and, thrillingly, now in South Africa, where we're tackling AIDS care, and in Malawi, where we're fighting maternal and infant mortality. I'm so grateful to so many of you in this room, and I just wish I had time to name all of our projects, and all of you.

But I don't. I have to focus down largely on only one piece of all of this amazing work—a big piece, but only one piece—the Campaign. My main job in this speech is to launch the successor to the 100,000 Lives

Campaign. Forgive me for being so focused. I know how much else is happening, and I love it.

But, let's start with Paul Cézanne.

He was, of course, the great French impressionist. He left his native Provence for Paris in 1861, when he was twenty-two years old, but his heart stayed in Provence, and he spent the last two decades of his life there.

Cézanne apparently was a bit of a grouch. But, he could paint. I don't know much about art, but even I know what Paul Cézanne could do with a brush, and paint, and canvas. He painted apples that you want to touch, textiles that look like mysteries, and faces that are maps of souls.

This summer, I went to the exhibit called *Cézanne in Provence* at the National Gallery in Washington, D.C. And I came to a wall there that I won't ever forget. Cézanne, like Monet, painted certain motifs over and over again. He didn't paint apples once; he painted them hundreds of times. But another motif that appears all through his career is a mountain, Mont Sainte-Victoire. It's in Provence, within sight of his birthplace. He painted it more than sixty times. The last time was the week he died, at age sixty-seven.

In 1902, when he was sixty-three, Cézanne set up his easel near his studio, and he painted Mont Sainte-Victoire from that exact same place— that very spot—not once, not twice, but twenty-eight times in the four years before he died—eleven oil paintings and seventeen watercolors. The exact same thing from the exact same spot twenty-eight times.

The exhibit in Washington had five of those eleven oils from around the world, and they hung all of them on a single wall, side by side. And, when I saw them there, on that wall, all together, I couldn't move. I started to cry.

Now, that's embarrassing: crying in public in front of a wall. I needed some help. So I called Dr. Terri Southgate; she's the editor who for thirty years has been choosing the *JAMA* cover page, which always has a work of art on it. I asked Terri why Paul Cézanne made me cry.

She said, "It's his honesty; it's his honesty in the face of nature." Cézanne respected nature, and he was trying to understand what he respected.

Claude Monet was different; he was a technician. His series on water lilies or haystacks are demonstrations; he's showing off what he can do. Monet's paintings are about Monet.

But Cézanne's images of Mont Sainte-Victoire aren't showing off; they're acts of reverence. He's more interested in knowing something, than in showing something. Terri thought it was Cézanne's respect that made me cry. He was trying and trying and trying to know. He wasn't going to give up—ever.

Look at his paintings. Look at the mountain: dark, light; glowing, withdrawn; distinct, vague; soft, stark. It's like Cézanne's asking, "Who are you? What are you? Why are you?" It's like Paul Cézanne found something more important than Paul Cézanne. He's sort of praying.

Think with me about the 100,000 Lives Campaign. It's been a wild two years since we announced it in 2004. Over three thousand hospitals joined. We visited hundreds of them, and we found more energy, more reach than I've ever seen before in health care. It's stunning—it's a new chapter.

So, now I get to announce the next Campaign—where I hope we can go—what I hope we can do. But, first, I have a question. I am confused.

The Campaign contains a paradox. On the one hand, the Campaign demands standards. It asks people to pledge allegiance to science—to evidence. It asks them to line up straight, and to go after one, single, shared goal. It takes help; but it doesn't take votes. It says, in effect, "You don't have any choices—or, rather, you only get one choice: join, or don't join." That's up to you, but, once you're in, you're in; you're supposed to toe the line. If the science says, "Do it," then do it! The 100,000 Lives Campaign is a straightjacket. It's handcuffs.

And yet, look at what happened. Thousands and thousands of people—doctors, nurses, pharmacists, therapists, technicians, managers, executives—thousands said, "Okay, lock me up." They actually seemed to love it.

Here's a story. At last year's Forum, just after my opening speech, a woman—she said she was a nurse—came up to me. She took my hand, and she said, "I just want you to know that . . ." And then she started crying. She never finished the sentence. She just gave me a little wave, she smiled, shrugged, and she walked away. But, actually, she didn't have to finish her sentence. I knew what she wanted to say. She wanted to say that the Campaign added meaning to her life; that it added joy to her work. And she wanted to tell me that, for some considerable time before, those jewels—joy and meaning—hadn't been there for her. I know that's what she wanted to say because so many other people finished that sentence for her so many times to so many of my colleagues in these past two years.

But, hold on a minute! What went wrong at work? Well, I suspect it was handcuffs. Straightjackets. I think she felt accused, controlled, mistrusted, disrespected, misunderstood. She had been reading about pay for performance, as if she were a trained seal who jumped for fish. She had been reading about public report cards, as if she were a reluctant child. She had been reading about how her patients got hurt, as if she wanted to hurt them. She had seen doctors and nurses blamed severely for human errors that she knew, for sure, she, herself, would some day make—errors that, perhaps, she had made, secretly. She had seen the guidelines and rules in glossy manuals from insurance companies and outside reviewers that were supposed to be her roadmaps for care, never mind what she thought or knew. Her work day had become filled with mindless, silly record-keeping, so that she could write down all the things she wished she had time to do properly, if only she didn't have to waste time writing them all down.

She felt handcuffed. She felt trapped. Pride—joy—gone.

And that's the paradox. The Campaign isn't any different, is it? After all, it locks people up in a straightjacket of aims and rules—aims they didn't choose—rules they didn't make. Somebody else said, "Save one hundred thousand lives"—that nurse didn't. How did that tap pride and joy in the very same disheartened people who feel trapped by goals that they are ordered to pursue and by rules from strangers whom they have never met?

Why did that nurse cry with joy about a Campaign that locked her in? That's the paradox.

I don't really know why. I really don't, but I'll give it a shot in a few minutes. Maybe Paul Cézanne can help. But, first, I am going to make the problem even worse. I'm going to give you more rules, more handcuffs, a new straightjacket. Buckle up.

We are going to relaunch this—the next Campaign—right now. There's a basic framework that has five parts.

Part One of the Framework: The 100,000 Lives Campaign Isn't Over

It never will be. How could it be? Eliminating needless deaths isn't a restaurant bill; it's a utility bill; it's rent. The six Campaign planks are the new standard of work. We don't just need to make those changes; we need to maintain them. Like Nike says, "There is no finish line."

Part Two of the Framework: If You Were In, You Are In, Unless You Specifically Opt Out

For the thirty-one hundred hospitals who signed up for the 100,000 Lives Campaign, we're going to assume, for now, that you're in. You'll get to confirm this, or not. And, if you were in the first Campaign, don't worry; we're not introducing any new rules or confusing details.

Part Three of the Framework: New Goals—Reducing Injuries from Care

We'll keep working with you to end needless death. But now we're going to add another aim: to end needless pain and suffering. We'll start with "No injuries from care."

Part Four of the Framework: Strengthening the Infrastructure

The 100,000 Lives Campaign wouldn't have had a prayer without so many key partners, beginning with Dennis O'Leary and the Joint Commission on Accreditation of Healthcare Organizations, but including so many others—the American Medical Association; the American Nurses Association [ANA]; the Leapfrog Group; the National Quality Forum [NQF]; federal agencies like the Centers for Medicare & Medicaid Services [CMS], the Centers for Disease Control and Prevention [CDC], the Agency for Healthcare Research and Quality [AHRQ], and the Veterans Health Administration; and multihospital systems like VHA, Premier, SSM, Ascension, Allina, and Kaiser Permanente. All of that energy got leveraged through the Campaign's "Nodes," the leadership groups that came together and took responsibility for helping clusters of hospitals. The Node in Washington state, an alliance, got every single acute care hospital in that state into the Campaign. That simplified things. One call to that Node, and we were, in effect, contacting seventy-two hospitals all at once. The Association of American Medical Colleges [AAMC] was a Node; so were UHC, the National Rural Hospital Association, and the National Association of Public Hospitals and Health Systems.

This infrastructure—partners and Nodes—can be a new way to change at a national scale. I think it could be like a national rail system whose tracks can carry many different trains. We—IHI and our partners—will use those tracks, but others can, too, if we build the system right and if we strengthen it. And that's exactly what we're going to do.

That Leads Me to Part Five of the Framework: We'll Still Focus on Hospital Care

Now, that's been a very tough decision. Our email in-boxes are blazing with requests from around the nation—dreams—about new Campaigns.

How about a Campaign on mental illness? A Campaign on disparities? On prevention? On long-term care? Rural health? Public health? Chronic illness care?

We made a tough call: to keep this Campaign's focus, for now, on hospital care. That's where our sickest people lie; that's where so many tragedies happen; and the hospitals are asking us to keep going. In IHI as a whole, we do work across the continuum. All the cochairs of this National Forum—Doug Eby, Patty Gabow, Mats Bojestig, Sven-Olof Karlsson, and Göran Henriks—they all lead integrated systems, and that is not an accidental choice. But, today—here at the Forum—we're going to talk about hospitals.

Here's the goal: prevent injuries to patients in American hospitals over the next two years—twenty-four months. How many injuries? Five million. In the next twenty-four months, let's prevent five million incidents of needless pain and suffering—and needless deaths—that would have afflicted American hospital patients if we did not change care.

Let me show you how we get to that number. It involves a chain of logic, and a leap of faith.

The first step in the chain: How many hospital discharges are there in a year? The American Hospital Association [AHA] National Hospital Survey for 2005 says thirty-seven million.

The second step: How often are those patients harmed by their care? That's a harder question.

Brent James from Intermountain Health Care did a review of rates of harm from some of the best studies we have. He found that injuries from care occur in from 3 percent to 17 percent of patients.

How many injuries you find depends on how you go looking for them. The harder you look, the more you find. For years, IHI's R&D team on patient safety has looked very hard in dozens of hospitals. We classify the harm in the categories of the so-called NCC MERP system—the National Coordinating Council for Medication Error Reporting and Prevention. NCC MERP grades the severity of medication errors into nine levels: the least severe (Category A) to the most severe, death (Category I). We look for injuries of severity E through I.

Let me show you some real examples.

Category E are physical injuries from care that are temporary. They don't cause hospitalization or extend length of stay, but they do need monitoring or treatment.

Here is an example of an E injury: An elderly woman got started on antibiotics, but her care providers forgot that she was on an anticoagulant. She got an injection, and that caused a large and painful bleed into her thigh muscle.

Category F injuries are temporary, but they require a hospitalization for treatment or they prolong length of stay.

Here's an example: A retired farmer who had a hip replacement fell out of his hospital bed and dislocated his new hip. They took him back to the operating room to fix it, and he went home a few days late.

Category G injuries are permanent ones.

A fifty-nine-year-old man who had heart bypass surgery got a surgical site infection, and needed several additional operations and weeks of antibiotics. He was left with a markedly deformed chest. His harm is Category G.

Category H injuries require intervention within one hour to save the patient's life.

Here is an H: A sixty-four-year-old lung cancer patient had elective surgery. One hour after the surgery, the nurse found him unresponsive. He was resuscitated and brought to the operating room where they fixed a bleeding artery.

Category I injuries cause or contribute to death.

Here is an I: A fifty-five-year-old bus driver started on anticoagulation for atrial fibrillation. Three days later, he had a massive bleed into his brain—a stroke. He died six days later.

To find these injuries, we review hospital charts. A random sample of twenty charts a month is usually enough for a hospital to get a handle on its injury rates. Our team uses the IHI Global Trigger Tool to support those record reviews. Now, if your hospital is going to join the new Campaign, absolutely the best move you can make to get started is to look for injuries—to start that monthly search of twenty records every month. You can become expert searchers, but you'll have to put on new glasses—you'll have to change the way you search.

The Global Trigger Tool isn't perfect; but it's good enough for now. We've used it in dozens of hospitals, and here's what we find: in general, for every hundred admissions to a hospital, there are between forty and fifty injuries to patients. Actually, we've seen it as high as eighty. The cases I just talked about come from the actual reviews in one hospital that's famous for its safety results, and that hospital has a rate of forty-six injuries per hundred admissions after some of its best progress on safety. That is an astounding number—it's at least twice as high as rates you'll find generally published in journals. Why so high? For several reasons. Here are four:

- First, the IHI Global Trigger Tool includes injuries of Categories E through I. Lots of others start at Category F, and about 60 percent of E through I injuries are E.

- Second, the Global Trigger Tool is like a metal detector—it helps you focus your reviews, so that you can see the harms faster.

- Third, we don't distinguish between preventable and nonpreventable injuries. We think it's more modern to measure both. Prevent the ones we can with current knowledge, and always to try to figure out how to prevent more by getting smarter.

- And, fourth, we include some events that occur outside the hospital that cause the patient to have to be admitted; most others don't.

Here is the profile of events—preventable and nonpreventable—in one of the safest systems in the nation, LDS Hospital.

We are going to go with it—these findings. They'll be debated, they'll be criticized, and we'll deal with that as it comes. But, if we are right enough, and if you are willing to include Category E injuries as enemies, then we have a bogey: thirty-seven million admissions multiplied by, at the low end, forty injuries per hundred admissions—that's fifteen million injuries per year in American hospitals. That's the third link in the logic chain.

Our goal—the goal for this Campaign—the leap of faith—is to stop 5 million of those injuries over two years—2.5 million a year—2.5 million of the annual 15 million injuries. That means an average improvement in patient safety of 2.5 million divided by 15 million, or one-sixth—17 percent.

We're going to call it the "5 Million Lives Campaign." Actually, some injured patients get injured more than once, so preventing five million injuries is not quite helping five million different people. But, for simplicity, we're going to call it the 5 Million Lives Campaign, knowing that sometimes we'll be counting the same person—the same life—twice. Obviously, also, in this Campaign, "lives" means something different. Sometimes it's still "lives saved," but more often now it's "lives bettered," "lives unharmed," or "safer lives."

Of course, we're not going to be 17 percent safer on day one. We'll have to ramp up. And, if we want to ramp up steadily over two years, and still have injuries be five million fewer two years from now, we're going to have to reach a state twice as safe as that by the very last day of this two-year Campaign. Oh, my goodness! To save five million injuries, we need to be two-times-17 percent—or 34 percent—safer two years from now, on December 12, 2008, at 9:00 a.m. Eastern Standard Time—all over America, in every hospital. One-third of health care injuries gone, in just two years.

Incredibly, even that won't make care safe—we'll still have a long way to go. But, it will be massive. The 5 Million Lives Campaign is going to try to chalk up the largest improvement in patient safety in American health care history.

Some is not a number; soon is not a time. Five million better lives; December 12, 2008, 9:00 a.m.

How? Let's start where the payoff is. The research helps us to focus down on five specific forms of harm—a starter set where the 5 Million Lives Campaign can begin, but can't end.

1. Prevent Pressure Ulcers

I don't know if you have ever seen a pressure ulcer. I have; my father had one. They have four stages: red skin, a blister, a full-fledged sore, and a sore that goes right through the entire layer of skin. They're ugly, painful, hard to treat, and they can kill you. And almost every pressure sore is preventable. We know that from science, and we know that from pioneers.

One of those pioneers is the Ascension Health hospital system—three years ago, led by Ascension Health nursing, they declared "war on pressure ulcers," and they're winning the war. Rates in Ascension's sixty-seven hospitals are 90 percent lower than the US average; they're just over one per one thousand bed days. Now, you go there, too. How do you prevent a pressure sore? We've worked with Ascension, with the Nursing Home Quality Campaign, and with scientists who've been tackling this problem for a decade, and we will give you the rule base—your new straightjacket—a pressure sore "bundle" that's your lever for eliminating this scourge. It's too late for my father, but maybe not for yours.

2. Prevent MRSA Infections

Methicillin-resistant *Staphylococcus aureus* [MRSA] infections are about as close to a doomsday bug as we ever want to get. The problem is epidemic, and it's expensive. Half of MRSA infections are picked up in the hospital. They're not inevitable. They can be prevented, maybe even eliminated. I visited Ryhov County Hospital in Jönköping, Sweden, last spring. Guess how many cases of MRSA their patients get a year. The answer is zero—never even one. International variation is extraordinary—resistance rates from practically zero in Denmark and the Netherlands to 45 percent in England. "Every system is perfectly designed to get exactly the results it gets." What system has a resistance rate of zero and what system has 45 percent? I want to thank CDC, the Society for Hospital Epidemiology of America, the Association for Professionals in Infection Control and Epidemiology, and other great colleagues in the nation's infection control community; they've been working hard with us on this plank. Thanks largely to them, we now have a first-draft strategy for hospitals to prevent—maybe even eliminate—MRSA.

I need to give a shout-out to the Illinois Hospital Association. They already heard about this MRSA goal, and they say they want to be the nation's leader in results. Get going, or I think you'll be watching their tailpipe. How about a derby? Who wants to try to beat Illinois? VHA has also just announced a massive MRSA campaign.

3. Eliminate Injuries from High-Alert Medications

They are anticoagulants, sedatives, narcotics, and insulin. Of the fifteen million per year E though I injuries, we find that 50 percent are due to drugs, and 58 percent of those are due to high-alert medications. Do the math: that's over four million high-alert medication injuries per year. The 5 Million Lives Campaign will ask you to focus on those culprits.

4. Reduce Complications of Surgery by Adopting SCIP

The Surgical Care Improvement Program [SCIP] was started by CMS and embraced by a long list of partners, including the American College of Surgeons, CDC, the AHA, IHI, and others. SCIP aims to reduce surgical complications, which happen in 40 percent of the forty-two million inpatient and outpatient operations in the US each year, by three hundred thousand a year—25 percent by 2010—in Medicare patients, alone. It's time to make SCIP the American standard, everywhere, and I think the Campaign can offer some railroad tracks for that train.

5. Make the Care of Congestive Heart Failure Reliable— Utterly Reliable

Five million Americans have congestive heart failure [CHF]; it causes a million hospitalizations a year. It's the most common reason for admission in Medicare. The 14 percent of Medicare beneficiaries who have

CHF account for 43 percent of Medicare costs. Flaws in CHF management are rampant. The consequences in complications are big—prolonged hospital stays, increased disability, and "bounces"—readmissions. In 2005, Medicare patients had 616,000 discharges with CHF. Of them, 17 percent bounced in fifteen days; 27 percent in thirty days; and 39 percent in sixty days. Those failure rates are unnecessary. One landmark study by Fonarow and colleagues, published by the *Journal of the American College of Cardiology* in 1997, showed how to decrease rehospitalization rates by 85 percent. With CHF, we propose that the best care should be the standard of care. Our scientific colleagues in this include CMS, the Joint Commission, the American Heart Association, the American College of Cardiology, and the Society for Hospital Medicine.

In the 5 Million Lives Campaign, we're also going to add one more plank—a different kind of plank. We call it "Boards on Board." It's a call for hospital boards to accept direct responsibility for reducing patient injuries.

I want to speak directly to board members and executives for a minute, if you can hear me. I want to be a little pushy. We need to think differently about the job of governance in health care. Here's the new way to think. Let's say MRSA infections are avoidable (and they are), and let's say board action is a precondition to the necessary investments to prevent those infections (and it is), and let's say a board fails to do its part to go after that goal. Then, couldn't someone allege that that hospital board is at least partially responsible for the MRSA infections in that hospital? This is an era of increasing corporate accountability. Don't be surprised if some begin to assert that boards that don't help stop avoidable injuries are partly responsible for those injuries. Here's a happier way to think about it: if pressure sores, surgical complications, and injuries from high-hazard medications can be prevented, then boards that insist on that prevention have a wonderful opportunity—they can actively help protect their patients from harm.

One of IHI's first board members, Jim Bakken, used to tell me that boards are not seats of honor; they are positions of responsibility, and that includes responsibility for the continual improvement of care. Let's declare 2007 in health care to be the Year of Governance.

And so, the sixth plank in the 5 Million Lives Campaign is this.

6. Get "Boards on Board"

I think boards will welcome that challenge; they don't want to be AWOL on patient injuries. They want to check in, but they need help. We have lots of great examples already of boards that are engaged in patient safety as a priority in novel and energetic ways—for example, at Cincinnati Children's Hospital Medical Center, at Virginia Mason, and at Exempla. These give us all models, and drawing on those models and others, the 5 Million Lives Campaign will help. We'll offer specific advice for any willing board about how they can reduce patient injuries.

These are our new enemies: pressure sores, MRSA, harm from hazardous medications, unreliable care for CHF, and surgical complications. And, we add one more: a raised bar for boards.

These targets won't be enough to stop five million injuries over two years—not nearly enough. They account for too few injuries to get us there. So this 5 Million Lives Campaign has one other, crucial, element: your space. The "plus" space. Even more than in the 100,000 Lives Campaign, we're going to exhort hospitals all over the country to add their own changes—your own improvements—to share them with us, and let us share them with the nation. These are a starter set. You can find more; just look. You can start with the terrific organizations in the United States already working hard on patient safety: the National Patient Safety Foundation, the Institute for Safe Medication Practice, CMS, our amazing Quality Improvement Organizations [QIOs] and the American Health Quality Association, AHRQ, Leapfrog, the Joint Commission, ANA's National Database of Nursing Quality Indicators, the National Business Group on Health, NQF, Consumers Advancing Patient Safety, and dozens more. We are aligned with the American Heart Association's "Get With the Guidelines" program. Boards can get help from the American Hospital Association's leadership center, the National Center for Healthcare Leadership, Estes Park Institute, and the Governance Institute. Canada is already out ahead with its national "Safer Healthcare Now" initiative. And the World Health Organization Patient Safety Alliance has launched its wonderful "High Fives" campaign in seven nations. If you dig, you're going to find gold.

Let me be perfectly clear. We are not saying for a minute that the 5 Million Lives Campaign is going to reduce injuries all by itself. That would be such a waste. There's a decade of work under our belts in this country to try to make care safer. NPSF, CMS, the QIOs, and that long, long list of helpers and pushers—that's a big investment in that job. What we are saying is that it is high time for a national return on that investment—high time to leverage that investment. The 5 Million Lives Campaign is not a replacement; it's a lever. Together—not separately—we can get our country to that goal. We can stop so much pain. And, when we succeed, "we" will mean "all of us." It will not be the Campaign that has succeeded; not the IHI that has succeeded; it will be our nation that has succeeded. There will be plenty of credit to go around.

The support has begun. I am thrilled that America's Blue Cross and Blue Shield health plans agreed to take on principal sponsorship of this new Campaign. I am deeply grateful to Cleve Killingsworth, president and CEO of Blue Cross Blue Shield of Massachusetts, and Scott Serota, of the Blue Cross Blue Shield Association, for their leadership in bringing this funding arrangement together—and John Fallon of Blue Cross Blue Shield of Massachusetts, who is here at the National Forum.

When we announced the initiative, the Cardinal Health Foundation—key supporters in the 100,000 Lives Campaign—were the first to offer help, and they did so at a level that elevates them to foundational partners for the 5 Million Lives Campaign. It's a tremendous boost toward our goal of being able to offer rich resources, expert knowledge, and targeted help across the country at absolutely no cost to participants.

We also have firm endorsements of the 5 Million Lives Campaign already from organizations representing thousands of hospitals: Premier, Kaiser Permanente, Bon Secours, Ascension, Providence, Exempla, the entire Veterans Health Administration, and more. And, from associations and agencies, like AAMC, AHRQ, and on and on.

When we announced the 100,000 Lives Campaign in December 2004, I was lucky to share this very stage at IHI's National Forum with some of the most respected leaders in American health care. A number of those same people and organizations are here at the Forum, joined by a few welcome new faces: Paul Schyve, senior vice president of the Joint Commission on Accreditation of Healthcare Organizations; Becky Patton, president of the American Nurses Association; Steve Mayfield, vice president of the American Hospital Association; Rusty Holman, president elect of the Society for Hospital Medicine; Steve Jencks, from the Centers for Medicare & Medicaid Services, and a senior fellow at IHI; David Pryor, senior vice president of Ascension Health; Sister Mary Jean Ryan, chief executive officer of SSM Health Care; Sorrel King, of the Josie King Foundation; and Dr. Julie Gerberding, director of CDC. Each of these friends is already a patient safety leader, and it's an honor to have them here.

Is this going to work? I didn't know when we launched the 100,000 Lives Campaign, and I don't know now. Believe me, this 5 Million Lives Campaign is going to be much tougher. Measurement is tougher. Transparency is tougher. The cultural changes are tougher. We'll have to learn how to apologize, as Lucian Leape is saying we need to. And the science is tougher.

Safety science is uncompromising. Many of the changes in care are hard—harder than the 100,000 Lives Campaign planks. They're straight-jackets. I think MRSA is nearly eradicable, but only if hand washing becomes as inevitable as breathing. No one has cracked that nut yet. The SCIP changes require total teamwork. High-alert medications need to be handled like dynamite. Pressure sores are highly sensitive to nursing practices, and you can't implement them reliably unless nurses have the support—the time, equipment, skills, and ergonomic safety—to do their work properly.

To make care safe, we need more help from patients and families. We need their knowledge and vision, and we need them to increase their impatience. They have a right to breathe clean air, to walk safe streets, and to drink pure water. And they have an equal right to health care unpolluted by needless pain. Not a bone in my body believes that health care workers—doctors, nurses, others—cause injuries. Hardly ever is that meaningfully the case. So many people are trying right now, all over the country, to make health care safer, and they just can't succeed unless they have systems that help them succeed. It is the systems they work in—the designs—that trap them in defects they do not want to cause. But, to say that harm comes from systems doesn't excuse the harm. The time for patients to give us permission to have systems that can harm them is at an end.

Is this good news, or bad news? Are the handcuffs—this commitment to excellence—too tight? The nurse who cried—maybe she is here today—what is she thinking, feeling, now? Is she crying again for joy? Or, is she crying for a different reason?

Art experts call Cézanne's mountain—Mont Sainte-Victoire—a motif. A motif is what the world hands the artist: the thing, itself. Terri South-gate says Cézanne was "an absolute servant to nature. . . . What always struck me about him was his humility in front of nature."

This 5 Million Lives Campaign does not have to be a prison. It is—it ought to be—art, but art as Cézanne loved art; art with humility in front of nature. We did not choose the laws of science any more than Cézanne built Mont Sainte-Victoire. The biochemisty of MRSA; the importance of hand washing; the microcirculation of the skin; the dynamics of blood clots and peptic ulcers—these aren't ours to choose. Honoring our patients, honoring our better selves, means honoring nature and respecting her laws.

Embracing autonomy is no excuse to ignore nature. We know better than that. Why agree to absolute reliability? To standards? To ending senseless variation in our care? Why wash our hands? Not because we are robots, but because we respect nature.

And then, of course, the art begins. That's the secret of the Campaign. Every one of us is Cézanne. We stand before the mountain—nature; we bow—servants to truth; and then, we paint. Our own lives and our day-to-day work are our canvas, and our imaginations are the colors. We follow the rules; but we make them our own, our own way. That is what the poet does who chooses to write a sonnet in fourteen lines. That is what a composer does who writes by the same rules of harmony that Mozart did. And that is what a doctor, or nurse, or pharmacist, or therapist does who insists on better systems that reliably turn knowing into healing.

But, something's still wrong with this picture, and I know it. As the clock ticked toward this speech—the launch of the Campaign—I didn't sleep well. And, I'll bet you're not so comfortable, either. Five million injuries? Thirty-four percent improvement? Have we lost our minds? I want to galvanize you, but I don't want to electrocute you.

Let me tell you a secret. I grew up in a very small town—Moodus, Connecticut. My graduating high school class had fifty-three people in it. Everybody in Moodus knew everybody else.

I wasn't a very good athlete, but I tried. I was on the junior varsity basketball team in tenth grade. I was second string, and rarely got to play in a game. And, I had never scored a basket. Then, my chance came. The coach put me in, and I was psyched. I remember the moment—I was in the clear, I yelled for the ball, it came, I saw the basket. Incredibly, it was wide open. My heart raced. I drove for it, and I scored. I scored. For the wrong team. It was the wrong basket. To this day, I don't know how it happened. But it did happen, in full view of five hundred classmates and parents, in a very small town. I spent the rest of that game—which lasted ten thousand years—praying to God that we would lose by more than two points.

It's supposed to be funny now. It's so trivial compared to, say, patient safety. I am supposed to laugh. But, I am not laughing. Gertrude Stein said, "Inside, we are always the same age." Inside, I am still fifteen years old. I still feel my heart race as I take that shot. I still hear my teammate, Eddie, bewildering me with his screaming, "No, no, no . . . !" I still, in the middle of the night, suddenly, again, realize what I had done. I still remember my father's innocent question when I came home that night. He asked, "How could you have done that?" It's not funny. At age fifteen, or at sixty remembering fifteen, there aren't a lot of things less funny.

As an adult, I kept this a secret. I didn't ever talk about it until, for some reason, this year I finally told a journalist who was writing a personal profile on me. I don't know why I told him. But, I am telling you, too.

My guilt, my embarrassment—these could isolate me. But, as I wrote this speech, actually with the advice of my wise friend, Davis Balestracci, I suddenly realized something. Maybe it's the opposite. Maybe these connect us. I think, maybe, you, too, have your secrets. You tried, and tried, and tried. You finally got your chance, you found your courage, you saw the basket, drove for it hard, with all of your might, shot, hoping—and you were wrong, totally wrong, failed, embarrassed . . . human . . . in public. And, maybe, you hurt, too.

Paul Cézanne destroyed many more paintings than he saved. He would try, and destroy, try, and destroy, try, and destroy. Never, never, never—in his own view of himself—quite good enough. I could see that in his endless pursuit of Mont Sainte-Victoire.

And, here I stand—holding the ball again—wondering, inside, should I take the shot? What are we to do, you and I? We, with secrets about failing? We are here to help others. That is a very hard game to play, and we are already trying as hard as we can already. Five million people! Five million people with needless infections, and needless sores, and needless swollen arms, and aching skin, and trouble breathing, and bleeding, and fear, and, even, needless death. What are we to do? Take the shot? Or, not? My heart races, again.

I'm saying, "Take it." Let's stop five million harms in two years. Let's try to do something bigger than we have ever tried before. Let's aim for a goal so bold that we quake at its apparent impossibility.

No wonder some won't try. Even the name of our goal, "5 Million Lives," is enough to stop some. They don't want to take the risk; they remember the pain of failing. It was C. S. Lewis who said, "Courage is not simply one of the virtues, but the form of every virtue at the testing point." The virtue that we signed onto when we chose this field is the complete commitment to do whatever we can to relieve suffering, and the form it takes at the testing point is courage. Not the courage to conquer the enemies outside; but the courage to overcome the fear inside. Yes, I scored a basket for the wrong team; and, yes, I will try to help prevent needless pain—five million times in the next two years. And, if I fail, I fail. And if we fail, we fail. It is that simple. It's not courage if it can't fail.

The 100,000 Lives Campaign has had its share of critics, and the 5 Million Lives Campaign will have more. It's bigger and bolder, and it will draw more heat. Some may say that we overestimate our effects. That doesn't scare me, because we don't claim that the Campaign is alone. We'll ask only if the nation is safer. Some may question the scientific rigor of the changes we recommend. That doesn't scare me, because scrutiny is good, and because we are working with other groups who study the science, and because we are always ready—avid—to learn when better science emerges. Some may question our taking action when we aren't totally certain, when we only suspect strongly that we can help. That doesn't scare me, because I think that when the status quo is hurting people, getting change started is the right thing to do, and because I know that we can learn from what we do.

Questions don't scare me; cynics do. And, worst of all, our own cynicism, our own hopelessness, our own surrender to what goes wrong and should not go wrong. What scares me is the loss of our confidence that we are both smart enough to learn better how to help, and good enough to want to try.

Eleanor Roosevelt said, "You must do the thing you think you cannot do." Cynics won't. The fearful won't. The hopeless won't. But that is what the 5 Million Lives Campaign is doing—is asking—exactly. Put down your cynicism. Put down your fear. Put down your hopelessness. Pick up hope, knowledge, and trust in what you can do, and in what you can learn to do, as long as we do it together. Do the thing you think you cannot do.

I want you to stop harm. Today, there lies a man, seventy-five. Next week he'll have a sore on his back a half-inch deep. It will hurt him. It may kill him. Stop it. MRSA lies in wait to kill that young mother. Stop it. A blood clot is forming deep in a pelvic vein of that mother who's nearly better from her auto accident; it's aimed at her pulmonary artery. Stop it. That syringe has ten times the right dose of morphine inside. Stop it. No . . . no . . . that's too much coumadin; that artery—there!—in the brain!—it will leak the day after tomorrow, and that grandfather won't ever again be able to speak to his grandson. Stop it. Stop it.

Cézanne had his mountain; your motif is stopping needless pain. The causes are real. They are truth. You cannot change them. You must respect them. There are rules. You must honor the rules. The mountain is not yours; but, your palette is all yours. Each organization, each person in this room will, or will not—the choice is totally yours—place the easel of your work where you can see nature. And then you will, or you will not—the choice is totally yours—paint. And that is why the nurse cried. She cried because, at last, she was invited to paint.

Pick up your brush. Without nature, your paintings have no power. But unless you paint, nature lies unknown. With both, you and I stand, perhaps, with Paul Cézanne before the mountain—nature, we bow, and we cry a bit with joy at the possibilities.

FURTHER READING

Fonarow GC, Stevenson LW, Walden JA, et al. Impact of a comprehensive heart failure management program on hospital readmission and functional status of patients with advanced heart failure. *J Am Coll Cardiol.* 1997 Sep;30(3):725–732.

Chapter 5

A MESSAGE FOR RAMESH

COMMENTARY

Paul Farmer

WHAT IS THE greatest challenge before us as people involved
in providing effective and humane health care? Is it a
technical one, to be identified and elevated within some realm
of expertise, such as health policy or health care financing or
patient safety? Or is it more likely to be found in the messy,
painful process of thinking hard about what it means to be
human and humane? In this address, given to the young
graduates of an American university (and before the kin and
friends and teachers who have nourished and cared for them),
Don Berwick reminds us that it is the latter. Although
technical challenges abound in medicine and public health,
the ranking problem of any profession seeking to reduce
human suffering is the problem of disparities of risk and of
redress. These disparities constitute the great drama of
modernity: the chasm between rich and poor, well and sick,
self and other, fortunate and unlucky, protected and exposed,
oblivious and aware.

As in all of his speeches, whether to an audience unfamiliar
with the mortal drama of illness and privation or to those
steeped in its complexities, Don Berwick signals the urgency
and pathos of a wounded world. This is not always easy to
do. But he also invites his audience to play a role in repairing

it. His method, here, is to *engage* those spared (by good
fortune as much as by their own or their parents' industry)
privation in the grand project of addressing it. Don is not
trying to win an argument, but rather to open up a window
on the world as it is, while exhorting us to close the one
giving onto the trompe l'oeil world as we choose to see it.

To convey such a weighty message in a commencement
speech is no mean feat, and Don's approach, which has also
served him well among his professional colleagues and peers,
is to tell a story. This could be a story about what it's like to
be sick and poor, or injured and alone, or the victim of
serious medical error. Don has told these sorts of stories
before, of course, but they are probably not the best way to
bring a group of young Americans socialized for success into
reflection about their own position on a map of suffering that
stretches from Boston into its hospitals and clinics and
neighborhoods and across an unequal world. The story is less
about Ramesh Kumar, a "street child" from Delhi, and more
about a young American recently graduated from college,
visiting a friend in India, and embarking on his medical
studies.

As a device, the story has some narrative drive: "On the
fourth day that I knew Ramesh Kumar," reports the
commencement speaker, "he asked me for some money."
Ramesh's mother was sick, he averred, and Berwick, having
seen others afflicted and unattended in that city, tells us of no
reason to doubt it. The young man from Harvard Medical
School lent the boy from Delhi 50 rupees, about $6, making
him promise to pay him back the next day. When Ramesh
didn't show, our narrator reports he went looking for him, "a
little angry," to give him a piece of his mind about lying to
friends. After this reportedly awkward exchange, Don
Berwick never saw "his" rupees or Ramesh Kumar again:
"Nevermore."

It could have easily been a story about a young
professional from Delhi and his or her own Ramesh Kumar
and might well have been were Berwick speaking there. The
story isn't about nationality; it's about disparities and about
pathologies of power. Whether or not those gathered at
Suffolk University believed that the young physician-in-

training would stoop to lecture, right there on the mean
streets of one of the world's largest slums, to a homeless waif
about values, they themselves were getting a piece of Don
Berwick's mind. It's the piece haunted by all the Ramesh
Kumars, those who've missed out on the chance for a home,
an education, the promise of decent medical care when they
or members of their families are sick. And although Don
promises to focus on only one thing, "the most important
thing," he recites, in the course of his story, a long list of facts
and figures about global poverty. If a billion people live on
less than $1 a day, the chances of preventing illness caused by
hunger and foul water and poverty, or even of building just
and equitable systems for them when they are sick, are
lessened.

Don Berwick has spent the past three decades trying to
build compassion and mercy and human solidarity into health
care. Some believe that such values cannot be built into
systems of care. They assert that caregiving, like caring itself,
is the province of the individuals working in our institutions,
whether these are clinics or hospitals or the development
agencies collecting the grim statistics Don shares in this
speech. But it is not so. Such values can be reflected not only
by providers—and Berwick has done as much as anyone to
remind us that most care is provided by families and others
beyond the walls of our clinics and hospitals—but also in the
institutions in which we try, and often fail, to do our jobs.

I write this reflection from a village in rural Rwanda. Ten
years ago, it was home to a hospital abandoned after the
1994 genocide that took one million lives in less than one
hundred days. Such settings may not have been at the
forefront of Don Berwick's mind as he emerged as a
champion for improvement of the dysfunctional health system
in the United States. But, as he tells the graduates of Suffolk
University, global health and social justice were very much a
piece of his mind. Here in Rwanda, the world's neglect is not
seen as benign. It's easy (and in most ways correct) to observe
that malicious intent was the real engine of the war and
genocide. That's why there is so much attention, here, to
self-reliance and to Rwandan-led efforts to promote
development and reduce poverty. And they're succeeding, as

anyone in this village would note if they'd been working here over the course of a decade.

But the health systems built here also strive, if not always successfully, to build equity and compassion into the very system of care. There are national programs to build community-based insurance, to push prevention and care out into the rural regions in which most Rwandans live, and to reach their Ramesh Kumars and their parents—especially their mothers—with services ranging from primary care to the treatment of AIDS and, to return to another theme of Don's, leukemia and chronic disease, including major mental illness. There are electronic medical records. Training programs are blossoming across the country. The spirit of improvement is alive and well, even in a rural district hospital.

These systemwide improvements are among the reasons that life expectancy has doubled in Rwanda between 2000 and 2011. Deaths due to AIDS, tuberculosis, malaria, and vaccine-preventable illnesses have plummeted, as have deaths during childbirth. These are some of the steepest declines in mortality ever documented anywhere and at any time.

But integrated prevention and care are not the same things as caring. The health system offers care providers, including the young Rwandan trainees who will make the same mistakes our Harvard Medical student did by lecturing a homeless boy about thrift and other virtues, the chance to be more effective. But its architects seek to offer them a chance to be more humane and compassionate, too.

Don's message, given in 2006 and thus before he himself ascended to a role in Washington, is that none of us can really afford to cultivate a lack of fellow-feeling. By any calculus, all of us, whether we hear or read a speech like this one or never learn to decipher the written word, will one day need effective care. Nor can we assume that others, including those who like him do have arcane expertise, will do this hard work for us. He reminds us not through exhortation or harangue, but through gentle suasion, that while some people don't have the choice of ignoring the hard surfaces of our planet, no one should choose to live in ignorance of others' suffering. All of us hope, as surely as we breathe, for tenderness and mercy when we are sick or frail or failing.

Berwick believes that all of us who might hear him or read him have a role to play in addressing the outrageous disparities that define our modernity.

If "hope is not a plan," neither are compassion and mercy a health care system. So what about Ramesh Kumar, who was not, in the tale told by Dr. Berwick about the young Don Berwick, either sick or failing? Do we, as systems thinkers, need to remember the experience of those who are not even yet our patients when there are so many who are, whether in an Indian metropolis or a Rwandan village or the American capital, already sick? Don gives us a piece of his mind by asserting that the answer, every time and in every place, is *yes we do*. We do need to learn from our failures, personal and professional, because a utopian and compassionate vision, like hope, can help to lead us forward toward a plan. Whether we use anodyne terms like *quality improvement* or more unsettling ones like *social justice*, we know we have a long way to go before we live in a world—one world, not three— in which we do right by those still left behind by progress. There's no easy fix, no technology, no prescription that will replace our search for Ramesh Kumar in order to express regret for past failures and to prevent the next instance or embodiment of these failures as sickness or as pain or as other forms of suffering. Don Berwick the visionary thought leader and architect of better systems is, after all, the same fellow who failed to understand the basic human rights of Ramesh Kumar the uncreditworthy street urchin.

We don't know where Ramesh is today, or whether or not he *is* at all. We do, however, still have Don Berwick with us, and we have cause to be grateful for his humility and confessions, just as we have cause to be grateful for his leadership and courage.

A MESSAGE FOR RAMESH

SUFFOLK UNIVERSITY GRADUATE SCHOOL
COMMENCEMENT ADDRESS
BOSTON, MASSACHUSETTS, MAY 20, 2006

I FEEL DEEPLY honored to share this wonderful day with you and your loved ones. It's an intimate time. Thanks for giving me a piece of it.

I was thinking back to my own graduations—high school, college, medical school—looking for hints about what to say to you. Gradually, I came to my senses. Every one of those involved a graduation speaker, and, for the life of me, I can't remember a single word that any one of them said. Not one word. Now, *that's* a hint.

I was tempted to give you a list. Like Polonius gives to his son, Laertes, as Laertes heads off for university, in Shakespeare's *Hamlet*. By my count, Polonius gives Laertes ten recommendations: "Neither a borrower nor a lender be," and eight more, leading up to "To thine own self be true." Ten is a good number of suggestions. Ten Commandments, right?

But, that's a stretch. My high school graduation speaker, by the way, was a radio talk show host on our local station, WTIC in Hartford, Connecticut, and his name was James Dull. I remember *that* because the local newspaper, the *Middletown Press*, the next day actually ran a headline that read—I kid you not—"Dull Graduation Speaker." That's absolutely all I can remember. Ten is too many pieces of advice.

I thought, maybe, seven. Surely you can remember seven pieces of advice. There are seven digits in a phone number. But, seven is taken. A best-seller by Steven Covey is called *The Seven Habits of Highly Effective People*. It has sold over ten million copies since it first came out in 1990.

Here they are: (1) Be proactive; (2) begin with the end in mind; (3) first things first; (4) think win-win; (5) seek first to understand, then to be understood; (6) synergize; and (7) sharpen the saw. But, you can't remember seven, can you? Look, be honest; you already forgot number one, didn't you? Just read the book.

Seven is already too many. But, Steven Covey just couldn't leave it at that, and so he published a book last year called *The Eighth Habit: From Effectiveness to Greatness*. Now, that's not right. Eight was already taken—by the United Nations. The UN adopted in the year 2000 eight "Millennium Development Goals"—things for the whole world to accomplish within fifteen years, by the year 2015—nine years from now. Let me read them to you—I'm going to need them in a minute.

1. Eradicate extreme hunger and poverty. Cut malnutrition and the proportion of people earning under $1 per day by 50 percent.

2. Achieve universal primary education.

3. Promote gender equality and empower women.

4. Reduce childhood mortality. Cut under-five death rates by two-thirds.

5. Improve maternal health. Cut maternal mortality by three-quarters.

6. Combat HIV/AIDS, malaria, and other diseases.

7. Ensure environmental stability. Cut by half the proportion of people without safe drinking water and sanitation.

8. Develop a global partnership for development. Reform aid and trade with special treatment for the poorest countries.

Uh oh . . . I can see. I lost you. Vacant stares. You're looking at your watches. Eight is too many. Anyway, aren't those the goals for the world, not for you?

My college graduation speaker, believe it or not, was the Shah of Iran—Mohammed Reza Shah Pahlavi. That was in 1968. I can't remember his list. I do know that he was thrown out in a revolution in 1979, and so he might not have been a highly effective person. He probably skipped a habit. Maybe he didn't sharpen his saw. I don't think you'd want his list, anyway. I don't.

Five is a smaller number than either seven or eight. Islam has five pillars. That's a list that serves a great religion well, when used appropriately.

I could go on, number by number, but it didn't take me very long to realize that there's only one number that can work—one number that stands even a little, tiny chance of your being able to remember what I said when you give *your* first graduation speech thirty years from now. That number is "one." I get to ask you to remember one thing. That's it. It's an awesome responsibility. I have to think of that one thing that you *have* to know. The one thing that will shape your life. You know—the most important thing.

But I got it. Here it is. Are you ready? Number one: Find Ramesh Kumar. Can you remember that? What do you think number two is? Right . . . there isn't any number two.

When I was in medical school, probably about the same age as many of you, a close friend of mine from college was special assistant to the US ambassador to India, Daniel Patrick Moynihan. My friend was living on the US embassy compound in New Delhi, and he invited me to visit him.

It's by far the most interesting trip I have ever taken, right up to now. India swept me away with its colors and smells and sounds. It challenged every sense. Go to India if you ever get the chance. I walked the streets of Delhi for day after day while my friend was at work in the embassy, and I saw the signs of a great civilization. It was also the first time I ever saw extreme poverty, like those the Millennium Development Goals mention—the $1-a-day kind of poverty. I walked along the streets noticing big cardboard boxes on a lot of sidewalks. It actually took me two days before I realized that the cardboard boxes were shelters—they were homes—people lived in them. On the third day, I was walking along, alone, and suddenly started crying for no apparent reason—no reason, that is, except for the suffering. The suffering.

That was about when I met Ramesh Kumar. He was maybe ten or eleven years old. He was a shoeshine boy, a street child, although he did mention his mother from time to time. Ramesh became my guide. For three more days, he met me in the morning—actually I didn't need to find him, he always found me—and for a few hours a day he walked me around the streets of Delhi showing me the sights: a museum, an old astronomical observatory, a market. And, he showed me his friends.

On our second day together, Ramesh and I walked past a few of his friends, and I noticed that one of them was quite sick. He had a fever, and was covered in sores from impetigo. You probably had impetigo when you were a baby—a strep infection of the skin. You got a little penicillin or some bacitracin ointment, and, poof!, it was gone. But this kid—maybe eleven like Ramesh—was covered in the sores, and, even though I was only a medical student, I knew he was in trouble—maybe headed for a bloodstream infection. It could kill him. By then, I knew an

Indian doctor and the name of her hospital, and I asked Ramesh to take the child and me there. Somehow, I found the doctor and I asked her if she could help the boy with impetigo. She got him admitted. That's the last I saw of him.

On the fourth day that I knew Ramesh Kumar, he asked me for some money. Fifty rupees—which was about $6 then. He said that his mother was sick, and he needed to borrow the money overnight. "Really, Ramesh," I said. "You want to borrow the money? That means you'll pay it back to me?" "Yes," Ramesh said. "I will pay you back. I promise it."

Ramesh wasn't there on the next day. He didn't meet me. I knew where he usually hung out, and so I went to find him. He was there. He jumped when I called his name.

"Ramesh," I said. "Where is my money?" He was silent. "Ramesh," I said, a little angry, "you said you would pay me back. Did you lie to me? You shouldn't lie to friends."

He ran away. Ramesh never said a word. He just turned around and ran away, back into the tiny alleys, past the cardboard boxes, out of my life, into my future—into today.

I need you to find Ramesh Kumar. I need you to give him a message for me. I need you to tell Ramesh this: "I am sorry, Ramesh. I made a very big mistake. That money, Ramesh, was not my money. It was your money. You didn't steal it. It was yours—all along."

I think Ramesh knew that. He knew his rights. Somewhere in his eleven-year-old mind he knew that 30 percent of the world goes to bed hungry every night, and that I do not. He knew that his friend might die of a disease that I can laugh at. He knew that, in the year I speak to you, one million children will die from malaria, which I need not fear, and that two million people will die of tuberculosis, which I need not fear, and that two million people will die of AIDS, which I need not fear. He knew polio, which I need not fear. He knew leprosy, which I need not fear. He knew dengue. He knew that one billion of the people in the world cannot have a glass of clean water. That 2.6 billion have no sanitation, and that thirty-nine hundred children die every day—150 while I am speaking to you—because they don't have sanitation and clean water. He knew that, of fifty-seven million deaths in the world in 2002, one in five would be a child less than five years old—one child every three seconds—and that two out of every three of these are preventable with the most basic of health services, which I had and he did not. He knew that simple vaccines—for measles, diphtheria, tetanus . . . diseases which I need not fear—kill between two and three million children every year.

He knew that he was a little lucky because he got to be eleven years old. He knew that five hundred thousand women die of pregnancy-related causes every year. In Canada, the rate is one woman in eighty-seven hundred. In Nigeria, it is one in eighteen. He knew that a child born in India will live fourteen fewer years than my child in the United States. That a child born in Burkina Faso will live thirty-five fewer years than my child. That a child born in Zambia today has a lower chance of surviving to age thirty than a child born in England and Wales in 1840.

He knew that one billion people call mud a floor and sometimes even cardboard a roof. He knew that 21 percent of the world's population, over one billion people, live in extreme poverty—less a $1 a day—and that another 1.5 billion live on $1 to $2 a day. That the richest 20 percent of people in the world have 75 percent of the income, while the poorest 40 percent have 5 percent of the income. The combined income of *Forbes* magazine's five hundred richest people in the world exceeds the total income of the 416 million poorest people in the world.

Ramesh knew that that is not right. He knew that the 50 rupees, somehow, connected to all of this, and that—no matter what the laws of the rich say or the principles of the allegedly just—those 50 rupees were just as much his as mine. His problem was not to figure out whether he *should* have them; it was simply, solely, self-evidently to figure out how to *get* them. One billion people on this planet live on less than $1 a day. What do you think they are thinking?

Do you remember those Millennium Development Goals I told you about before—the eight goals? Of course, you don't. Eight is too big a number. But let me give you a status report, anyway. The goals were launched in the year 2000, and they are due for delivery in the year 2015. Last year, the UN reported on the progress worldwide. We're going to miss them—by a mile. The world promised, and then it didn't ante up. There were five targets for children by 2015: mortality, school enrollment, gender parity, access to water, access to sanitation. Instead of progress, fifty countries with nine hundred million people are going backward on at least one of those. Twenty-four of these are in sub-Saharan Africa. Sixty-five more countries with 1.2 billion people won't hit targets until after 2040—twenty-five years late. Because of this gap, forty-one million children are going to die by 2015 who would not have died if we had reached the goal. At the current rate of progress, sub-Saharan Africa won't reach its target death rate reduction until the year 2115—they are running a century behind schedule.

What would it take? The so-called Monterrey Consensus, under the auspices of the UN, in 2002, signed by the United States, re-ratified a

UN agreement signed in 1970—thirty-five years ago—that called for the wealthy countries of the world to commit seven-tenths of 1 percent of their gross domestic product each year to development assistance for the poor nations—for the Millennium Development Goals. Seven-tenths of 1 percent to end the devastation of extreme poverty. End it. When you make $100,000 a year, that will mean $700. In 2005, only five countries on Earth met that goal: Norway, Sweden, Denmark, the Netherlands, and Luxembourg. The United States gave, not seven-tenths of a percent, but two-tenths of a percent—the lowest of twenty-two OECD [Organisation for Economic Co-operation and Development] nations, except for Portugal.

Did Ramesh Kumar run away from his new American friend in shame? Was he embarrassed to be caught a thief? I don't know. I nevermore saw him at all. But, I will tell you, now thirty-three years later, the shame, Ramesh, is not yours; it is mine. Do not be embarrassed for yourself, Ramesh—be embarrassed for me.

I don't remember even the name of my medical school graduation speaker, nor a single lesson he or she told me. Not one. But I will remember until the day I die, with the vividness of the moment it happened, with the smells and sounds and colors of Delhi swirling around me, Ramesh Kumar running, and my immediate surge of anger, and then my deep and utter shame.

Where did he go? Where is Ramesh Kumar now? I shudder to imagine. He would be almost fifty years of age, if he ever got to fifteen.

Forty-three years ago, on the steps of the Lincoln Memorial, Martin Luther King called the United States Constitution a "promissory note" guaranteeing freedom and justice for all. He said that successive governments had issued for African Americans "a bad check which has come back 'insufficient funds.' . . . But," Dr. King also said, "we refuse to believe that there are insufficient funds in the great vaults of opportunities of this nation."

Today, it is not civil rights that involves a promissory note, it is human rights, and it is not the US Constitution that makes the promise, it is—it has to be—humanity itself. We have a bad check out there. Ramesh Kumar was just trying to recover what he had a right as a human being to have—safety, health, justice, a chance to grow, a chance to grow up, a chance not to have to be afraid of what the world has every chance to keep him from having to fear. Ramesh wanted what was his. Ramesh wants what *is* his. And I refuse to believe that there are insufficient funds in the great vaults of opportunity, compassion, and justice in the world to pay him what he is owed.

So, here is my one request for your graduation. Find Ramesh Kumar. He won't be that hard to find. He outnumbers you by a thousandfold. He is everywhere. He is billions. He is within a mile of this place—less. He is in the majority on almost every continent on Earth. And to find him, all you will need to do is to open your eyes.

Find Ramesh Kumar, and, when you do, tell him this for me: "I am sorry, Ramesh. It was yours all along."

Chapter 6

EATING SOUP
WITH A FORK

COMMENTARY

Paul B. Batalden, MD

IMAGINING HOW TO eat soup with a fork cleverly invites us to consider matching method and task. Developing a science of improving health care also requires that type of matching. When we use evidence to design and test a change for the improvement of health care, we follow a simple logic:

$$\text{Generalizable scientific knowledge} + \text{Particular context} \longrightarrow \text{Measurable performance improvement}$$

Each element of the formula represents a different knowledge system. We use different methods to build each knowledge system. For example, when we build generalizable scientific knowledge we carefully work to control "context" out as a variable. When we build knowledge of a particular context, we obsess about context and all we can learn about it—its processes, systems, habits, traditions, the things people celebrate, and so on. The methods we use, the questions we ask, are specific to the knowledge system we are using.

When we *make* an improvement, we are interested in questions like these:

- Why did you start?
- What assumptions did you make?

- What model of cause and effect did you have?
- What was the "work before the work" of making the intervention?
- What did you observe?
- What adaptations were necessary as you proceeded?
- What surprises did you encounter?
- What limitations might be important if others were to attempt to replicate what you did?

But *making* and *studying* improvements are two different tasks, with different types of questions and methods. In *making* an improvement we are subjects. We are actively engaged in assembling and connecting different knowledge systems. In *studying* an improvement we make an object of the improvement.

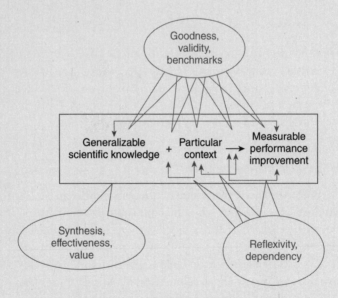

When we study improvements, we are interested in different questions, for example:

- What was your underlying theory or model?
- What methods of study did you use and why did you use them?
- What effects did you observe?

- What were the variations in effect, and what might have contributed to them?
- What inferences did you make?
- What analyses did you perform?
- What were the limitations of your study?
- What was your study context and what influences did it make on the intervention(s) being studied?

Jan Vandenbroucke, a student of clinical trials in the science of medicine, invites us to think clearly about the jobs of science and the importance of matching method with task. He notes that *science* is not the same as *evidence* or *assessment*, where a properly conducted randomized trial is a more powerful and a better-matched method than a case study. He suggests that another important function of science is *discovery* and *explanation*, where he reminds us that a well-documented case study is often more powerful and a better-matched method than a randomized trial.

Both making and studying improvement will be necessary to advance the science. Matching method, task, and question will be necessary for the development and advancement of a science of improving health care—another way of saying we need to know when to use a fork and when to use a spoon.

FURTHER READING

Vandenbroucke JP. Observational research, randomized trials, and two views of medical science. *PLoS Medicine*. 2008 Mar 11;5(3):e67.

EATING SOUP WITH A FORK

PLENARY ADDRESS
19TH ANNUAL NATIONAL FORUM ON QUALITY
IMPROVEMENT IN HEALTH CARE
ORLANDO, FLORIDA, DECEMBER 11, 2007

THIS IS MY nineteenth plenary address here. Each one scares me more. If you don't know what I mean, switch places and look out at seven thousand faces, and you'll get it. There are twice as many people here as in the town I grew up in.

So I prepare. I write the speech out and send it to IHI colleagues for comments. One of those this year was Joe McCannon, VP and head of our Campaigns. When he read my draft, Joe worded his advice carefully. He told me about a Bruce Springsteen concert that he once went to. Joe wrote, "At the start of the show, Bruce came out on stage and said, 'I'm worried that I'm going to make some of you unhappy tonight. I know that you'd probably like to hear some of my more well-known songs, but I don't think I'm going to play many songs you know tonight. I'm asking a lot of you. I know that. But I really think these new songs are important to play for you.' The audience was silent for about ten seconds," Joe wrote. "He wasn't kidding. They'd paid a lot of money. No 'Thunder Road'? No 'Born to Run'?" The story ends well. The audience forgave Bruce, and he played up a storm.

Now, what is Joe telling me? With advice like that, you have to read between the lines. Translation: "Don, this speech is a problem. People expect 'Thunder Road,' and this ain't it. Better warn them."

Now, I am not Bruce Springsteen—which strikes me as one of the least necessary sentences I have ever uttered. But, I *am* a little worried. This speech is not usual for me. It's wonky, and it's technical. I'm giving it because I think it is important, even if it's not what you expect. So, Bruce Springsteen and I now have one thing in common: I am going to ask a lot of you. If you're expecting "Born to Run," give it up.

If you don't get this year's Forum theme, "The Energy of Many," just look around. So many . . . doing so much.

We had our "Fall Harvest" last month for the 5 Million Lives Campaign. Nearly a hundred IHI staff—almost all of us—visited hospitals in all fifty states. We met hundreds of teams. They told us about what they were doing to fight infections, pressure sores, surgical complications, and a lot more. Our staff didn't need planes to get home; they were floating. The energy was electric.

I visited the University of Massachusetts Medical Center in Worcester. I got energy. Their cardiac cath team is reducing door-to-balloon times for heart attack victims—the ones for whom "time is muscle." First, a young pharmacist talked. The doctors, nurses, and managers stood at attention. Then, one by one, they explained their roles on the team. Their best door-to-balloon time so far is twelve minutes. Twelve minutes! They've cut their STEMI (ST segment elevation myocardial infarction) death rate in half. Just think of what's possible as the American College of Cardiology's terrific "D2B"—door-to-balloon—program, which now includes 975 hospitals and 38 partner organizations, gains traction.

We heard stories like that all through the Fall Harvest. Sure, we've got lots of work ahead in the Campaign. Measurement is tough. Getting into chronic illness care is tough. And, spreading change is tough. Some hospitals aren't getting results yet; some are stuck. They'll need more help.

And, it's a horse race. By the end of next year, Medicare says it will stop reimbursing hospitals for eight types of complication. In September, all of the hospitals in Minnesota decided to stop charging for twenty-seven "never events." Last month, the Massachusetts Hospital Association said its members will do the same for nine medical errors. And, just two weeks ago, Jon Perlin, the new chief medical officer for HCA, told me that all of the 178 hospitals in the HCA system will stop billing for never events.

The heat's on. We and our terrific allies in this Campaign work, the Joint Commission, the American Hospital Association, the American Nurses Association, the American Medical Association, the Leapfrog Group, and others, we know what we need to do now. We need to convert an episode—the Campaign—into a system, a national infrastructure for improvement. That's ahead. But, this is progress, and it is thrilling. It's fun.

Yet, there's a dark side—struggles, doubts. We get reminders that quality and safety problems aren't remote. They touch us.

I get a vivid window on this through my daughter Jessica, a third-year medical student now. She is sort of on a roller coaster. One day, she calls me, deeply moved by an encounter with a neonatologist teacher. He asked her, "What's the first thing you say to the parents of a premature newborn you admit to the ICU?" She thought, "We'll do everything we can for your baby." He said, "No. It's 'Congratulations.' "

That reminded me of my first afternoon with my clinical tutor, a surgeon named Dr. Ed Frank, in my first year of medical school. Dr. Frank brought me into Mrs. Smith's room—she had just had her gall bladder out. My first question was, "Where was your pain?" And then, I remember Dr. Frank's hand on my shoulder. He interrupted me. He said, "Don, do you know that Mrs. Smith has a brand new grandson?"

But, then, on another day, Jessica calls me, upset, to tell me about her friend, another student. In the operating room on his surgery rotation, he had been holding an instrument for hours, and his hand was cramping. When he couldn't stand it any longer, he asked the surgeon if someone could relieve him briefly. "I don't tolerate weakness in my operating room," the surgeon said. "The next time you complain will be the last time you operate with me." Through her tears, Jessica asked me, "What is *with* these people?"

I remembered a story that I told a few Forums ago, about a visit that my wife and I had to our obstetrician, Paul Goldstein, when Ann was pregnant with our second child. At the end of our visit, Paul asked us to stay a bit longer. "I know you're busy," he said, "but can I just ask you one more question? Today, in my office as my staff and I dealt with you, and as I examined you, Ann, and spoke with both of you, is there anything, anything at all, that could have gone better from your point of view?" And then, he sat back, quiet, just listening.

What's the difference? Why the whipsaw? What explains the excellence, the poetry, the loveliness of Paul Goldstein's question, Dr. Frank's guidance, that word, *Congratulations*? And what explains the distance, the harm, the indignity of that surgeon who calls human pain "weakness"? Is it parenting? Is it personality? Depression? Self-esteem?

The great Jewish philosopher, Martin Buber, says that human beings can adopt two different attitudes toward others: he calls them "I–It" and "I–Thou." *I–It* is how subjects relate to objects. People in *I–It* relationships see each other as parts—collections of isolated qualities. In *I–Thou* relationships, we see each other as whole beings. *I–It* relationships are detached; they have ulterior goals. *I–Thou* relationships are mutual; they are not a means to another end.

It isn't so hard to make the bad stories into good ones.

The surgeon could have said to the medical student holding the retractor, "I'm so sorry that you're in pain. Sometimes my hands hurt, too. Let's get you some relief. And, by the way," he could have asked, "did I do anything that made it hard for you to tell me sooner that you were in pain?"

To change a bad story into a good one, change it from *I–It* to *I–Thou*. Good stories aren't answers; they're questions. They're not about parts; they're about the whole. Not, "We'll do everything we can for your baby," but, first, "Congratulations."

There's a big difference between an *I–It* world of parts and an *I–Thou* world of people in complex relationships. When you are in one, but you yearn for the other, you can feel pain. You may have met this pain. I'm going to guess how. Here is the scene.

You're full of enthusiasm. You've studied the defects—say, infection rates, medication errors, delays in diagnosis. You know that there's a better way. You know that change is possible.

And so you put on your game face. And there you are in front of the medical staff. And you say, "Let's start some improvement projects. Let's nail it—the Ventilator Bundle, rapid response, better discharge planning. How about washing our hands?"

And, then the arm shoots up: Dr. Specialist, Dr. Respected, Dr. They-Named-the-Conference-Room-after-Me. And he says, "Very nice. But, where's the evidence? Where's the paper? Where's the clinical trial?"

Your face turns red. You need oxygen. You have flashbacks to that dream we all have in college where you show up for an exam in a course that you forgot to go to. You want to say, "Well . . . it just makes sense, doesn't it? Can't we give it a try?" But somehow, you know that won't quite do the trick. You're playing Quiddich, and the doctor just got the snitch. You're deflated. What the hell happened?

I'll tell you what happened. But, to find out, we have to go back in history, say, 120 years ago.

It's the early 1890s. Dr. William Halsted at Johns Hopkins University has a theory about how to fight breast cancer: radical mastectomy. Within a few years, it becomes the standard.

And, the Halsted Radical Mastectomy stays the standard for over eighty years. It prevails, even though there's no systematic evidence that it actually works. Then, in the 1960s, a few rather courageous cancer scholars, people like Dr. Bernard Fisher at the University of Pittsburgh, begin to study radical mastectomy with methods of formal evaluation that Halsted didn't know about. The most powerful method is the randomized clinical trial—the RCT, and *that* leads to a big surprise. According to RCTs, radical mastectomy is unnecessary. Survival isn't any better with it than with simpler forms of chemotherapy, radio-therapy, and breast-sparing surgery. Formal science shows that the emperor is naked.

This was an early skirmish in the battle for evidence-based medicine. The pioneers were people whose names you may not know: like Alvin Feinstein, Frederick Mosteller, Tom Chalmers, and David Sackett in the United States and Canada, and Sir Austin Bradford Hill, Archie Cochrane, and Ian Chalmers in the UK. They were tough; they had thick skin. They needed it. They were raising questions that traditional practitioners didn't welcome, and they used methods that medical schools didn't teach. They were iconoclasts, and the priests were unhappy.

But, they won. Evidence finally won. It took a while. But, by the mid-1980s we had a new taxonomy in the medical literature—a taxonomy of quality of evidence. It related the design of a study to the degree of confidence that could be placed on its findings. The lowest evidence was anecdote—the stuff of Halsted. The royalty of evidence was the randomized, prospective, double-blinded clinical trial. That's because an RCT done right could put more or less bulletproof protection around inference—protection against bias, confounding factors, self-delusion.

It was obvious. If radical mastectomy had been studied with an RCT sooner, tens of thousands of women would have been spared a disfigur-ing, painful, unnecessary procedure. Everybody realized that, when habits ruled, not facts, patients could get hurt. "Get out of storytelling," was the lesson; "Get into data."

So today, evidence-based medicine rules. We don't always have it, but evidence, especially randomized trial evidence, "Grade I" evidence, is what doctors learn to look for as the gold standard. With it, you can make your case. Without it, you can't. So, when Dr. They-Named-the-Conference-Room-after-Me raises his hand to question your puny PDSA cycle, he's been well taught. He doesn't want another Halsted procedure. He doesn't want stories; he wants facts. Good for him!

How do you get out of stories and into evidence? Get objective. Ques-tion beliefs; get the numbers; design the trials right; protect us against biases, against Halsted's misguided hopes. The randomized clinical trial is one of the greatest achievements of science in the twentieth century, because it makes inference *so* objective.

So what does Martin Buber—the *I–It* and the *I–Thou*—have to do with that? Maybe nothing. But, maybe something.

We in the room are agents of change. We're trying to get something new to happen in a very messy world. And . . . look at us now. Seven thousand people here. Twenty thousand connected. When we were a small group, it wasn't important that we could act. Now, it is. Isn't it only natural that people would wonder? Are we sure? Is this okay? Do we know enough? It is tempting to see the questions as attacks or resistance. Sometimes they are. It's easy to feel scared, doubting ourselves, and to slow down. But that doesn't feel right, either. There is another way. It's to meet the question on its own terms. How do we know? How can we learn? The tension is uncomfortable, but we can make it into an opportunity to mature.

Let's dive into an example: Rapid Response Teams. I first heard about these from Carol Haraden, when we were both visiting Australia about ten years ago. Carol had met Dr. Ken Hillman down there, and she saw some impressive results that Ken and his colleagues were getting with early response to patient deterioration. Ken had been an ICU director in Charing Cross Hospital in London a few years earlier. One night, a young woman came in with a broken femur from a bicycle accident. It all seemed routine. The orthopedic team put in a pin, and then, she died. Nobody expected it. Ken looked back, and he saw early warning signs that should have told the clinicians that trouble was brewing. But no one saw them or, if they did, no one did anything about them. What killed the patient, Ken says, were "silos of disengagement." Ken had a better idea.

Dr. Hillman shared with me a letter that I'd call historic. It's dated July 23, 1982, and, in it, he proposes to the head consultant in A&E [accident and emergency] at Charing Cross what may be the first clear description ever of a Rapid Response Team. Ken wrote, "This is a different concept to the cardiac arrest team. It is hoped that by providing earlier and more expert care, cardiopulmonary arrest may be avoided. The doctors called to seriously ill medical or surgical patients would provide rapid resuscitation and assessment." Ken knew—everybody knew—that a low percentage—only about 10 percent—of inpatients who arrest outside the ICU and are resuscitated survive to discharge. He knew also that many patients who arrest show early warning signs. Hillman's idea was logical: Don't wait for the arrest; anticipate it and act.

Before he had a chance to test his idea at Charing Cross, Hillman went back to Australia, to Liverpool Hospital. The doctors there at first rejected his idea for Medical Emergency Teams [METs]—they threatened their prerogatives. But finally, in 1989, Hillman got permission to study the MET system. His reports, mostly time series analyses, in the Australian literature, suggested great results.

So, Carol Haraden and I were impressed, and, back in the United States, our colleagues in the IHI—Carol, Roger Resar, Fran Griffin, Kathy Duncan, and others—began introducing rapid response to willing hospitals. Local reports began filtering back, and then flooding back, that the Rapid Response Teams did good—not always, but often. Hospitals told us that nursing staff felt less anxious, interdisciplinary teamwork improved, out-of-ICU cardiac arrests were less frequent, and, in some cases, even mortality rates fell. Not all hospitals were successful, and not all reports were dramatic, but the experience, as a whole, was positive.

So, when we launched the 100,000 Lives Campaign in December 2004, we included Rapid Response Teams as one of the six changes we called for. If *some* hospitals could make good use of it—and some *could*—we *knew* that—we thought that maybe *many* could.

Then came a hiccup—the June 18, 2005, issue of the *Lancet*—and the story of rapid response took a turn. There the research team that Ken Hillman, himself, had helped to form in Australia—the MERIT Study (Medical Early Response Intervention and Therapy Study)—reported on a cluster-randomized controlled trial of the MET system. Here is what the abstract of that paper said, in part: "The MET system greatly increases emergency team calling, but does not substantially affect the incidence of cardiac arrest, unplanned ICU admissions, or unexpected deaths."

Now, that's an oops! That's a collision! That's an evidence-based trump card. Forget the logic. Forget the intuition. Forget the stories, the celebrations, the local beliefs in local success. Forget what Ken Hillman thinks. We are caught red-handed. Halsted redux. Game over!

That's an overstatement, of course, but there were some strong words. If you were pushing for the 100,000 Lives Campaign in your own hospital, maybe you heard the echoes. Here are two examples:

From a team of health services researchers at Johns Hopkins University:

> "Given the equivocal evidence supporting the effectiveness of RRT programs, with the largest best-designed study showing no benefits, it is unclear why there is such interest in implementing this intervention and making it a care standard. . . ."

From a recent *New England Journal of Medicine* essay:

> "Early trials of medical emergency teams suggested a large potential benefit. . . . However, a large, randomized trial subsequently showed that medical emergency teams had no effect on patient outcomes."

I don't know how much this stuff chilled the work on early response, but it by no means extinguished it. Important consensus conferences focused on the topic, and they raised exciting, scholarly questions, inviting us all to think. For example, this one, from John Øvreveit, last August:

> Findings for one response team might not . . . be generalizable to other settings or over time, and . . . the intervention itself should continually evolve and improve. . . . An RRS (rapid response system) is not a drug treatment, a hospital is not a body. Both are continually changing, complex social interventions and cannot be understood through randomized controlled trials.

Meanwhile, the local work of thousands of hospitals in several nations continued to yield case-by-case results. We tracked them, and others did, too. We saw textured lessons about how and when rapid response designs of varying types appear to help, or not. Progress continued; but we *could* feel the discomfort.

I asked Ken Hillman this September what he really thinks. He told me what I already knew. The first point, and a major one, is clear to anyone who reviews the details of the *Lancet* study. It was *not* a negative trial. It was an *inconclusive* trial, not a negative one. This is because, despite the best efforts of this superb study team, it lacked statistical power, because there was cross-contamination between the treatment and control groups, and because the variation among hospitals was immense.

How do I know this? Well, I know it both from reading the study and from talking with the investigators. You see, they know the context. They know that making rapid response work well in any hospital isn't like taking a pill, like John Øvreveit says. It's like telling a story.

Let me take a liberty, with apologies to Martin Buber. What if it's true that learning how to make rapid response work isn't an *I–It* task? What if it's *I–Thou*? What if it isn't subject–object, but rather subject–subject? The stories about making rapid response work, after all, *are* pretty complicated ones. They're about leadership, and emotion, and changing environments, and details of implementation, and history. They're messy. A complex intervention—rapid response—experiences inevitable, complex variation in the details of its own mechanisms in local settings that, themselves, are textured, varying, and unstable. You see, a part of that story isn't the whole story—not by a long shot. That's the way it is with many system improvements—maybe even most. That's the way it is even with changes as apparently as simple as in the 5 Million Lives

Campaign. Why did I feel something thrilling as I stood in that corridor in the cardiac cath suite at UMass Medical Center, hearing a group of committed human beings telling me what they were trying, day after day, to do better and better for their patients. I didn't feel thrilled because it was simple. I felt thrilled because it was poetry.

There is something interesting—something sad—something costly—that, given the richness of the true story of rapid response, prestigious journals and capable scientific authors can write, "A large, randomized trial subsequently showed that medical emergency teams had no effect on patient outcomes." For the purposes these authors intend that contention, it is untrue. It is wrong.

Here is what I think is going on: I think that the improvement of health care in complex systems is both *I–It* and *I–Thou*. It is both about us and things and about us and each other. And, that means that, when we seek evidence, we are walking a tightrope. We need evidence, for the same reasons that Sir Austin Bradford Hill wanted evidence. We can't allow subjective hopes, wishes, and dreams to pretend to be truth when unforgiving nature is at work, or we will follow Halsted's error, and we will do harm. But the harm is equal if we treat a very complex world as if it were simple, if we treat each other as less than whole people and complex systems as simple and separate from us, and thereby reduce our capacity to learn, to converse, to explore, and to grow.

So, what *is* "evidence"? What is the new scholarship of improvement? The simplistic view is to consider objectivity as hard-headed and subjectivity as soft. It is to pit science against passion and belief against proof. That is not necessarily right. The opposite of science is not passion; it is ignorance. The opposite of passion is not science; it is torpor. When harm in the status quo is actively underway; when our relationship to what we study is deep and caring; when we can use all of our senses to acquire, not just data, but wisdom, and not just about parts, but about the whole; then we can be both passionate *and* scientific. Love and learning are not each other's natural enemies.

Health care tactics today are way over on the *I–It* side: pay for performance; jokes about herding cats; "In God we trust; all others bring data"; "If you can't measure it, you can't manage it"; the pursuit of accountability—each of these assumes or creates a dynamic between people as subjects and people as things. Themes from *I–Thou* sound different. They sound like this: curiosity; "There but for the grace of God go I"; storytelling; "continuous cycles of learning"; and, I think, Tom Nolan's recent breakthrough that he calls "Act with the individual; learn for the population." Or, as a colleague from Wales, Paul Buss, reminded me earlier this year in words from *The Little Prince*: "It is only with the heart that one can see rightly; what is essential is invisible to the eye."

Subject–object relationships are not bad. Linear evidence, hard, cold facts are necessary; we need them; our patients need us to have and use them.

I don't need to know who made my car; or who is flying my plane; or who designed the plane. That's a world of objects to me. It's all *I–It*. But, when I am in pain, or in fear, or confused, or at the end of my life—when I suffer—the person helping me matters in an entirely different way. In large measure, the relationship *is* the point. So, medicine, health care, health care improvement—these lie neither wholly in *I–It* nor wholly in *I–Thou*; we are creatures of both lands.

Two British social scientists, Ray Pawson and Nick Tilley, wrote a book called *Realistic Evaluation*. They help me think about what I will dare to call, fully admitting that it diminishes Buber's real message, *I–Thou* science—subject–subject science, as opposed to subject–object science. That's science that can still grow wisdom, with discipline, when systems are complex and when relationships matter. The science that knows that, in some important way, the heart *can* see what the eyes cannot.

Pawson and Tilley call the classical evaluation design "OXO." Observe a system—O; then perturb it—X; and then observe it again—O. The pinnacle for OXO evaluation is, of course, the randomized clinical trial. But, when you try to use OXO studies to evaluate results in complex systems, to evaluate social changes—and believe me, Rapid Response Teams are social changes—that's sort of my point—Pawson and Tilley find some serious limitations. In fact, OXO experimental evaluations of social programs almost always come up dry. OXO studies tend to conclude either that "nothing works" or, more often, that the results are inconsistent and therefore that "more research is needed." This is just about exactly where so many studies of quality improvement efforts in health care end up: studies of Rapid Response Teams, chronic disease management projects, or improvement Collaboratives, to take some recent examples. Time after time, the OXO researchers can't find the proof.

There are two possible conclusions from this boringly recurrent finding: either (a) nothing really *does* work usually, or (b) we are asking the wrong way. Here is what Pawson and Tilley say:

> For us, the experimental paradigm constitutes a heroic failure, promising so much and yet ending up in ironic anticlimax. The underlying

logic . . . seems meticulous, clear-headed and militarily precise, and
yet findings seem to emerge in a typically non-cumulative, low-impact,
prone-to-equivocation sort of way.

"The experimental paradigm constitutes a heroic failure." Whoa!
Have Pawson and Tilley called the whole evidence-based medicine
program on the carpet? Was Sir Austin Bradford Hill a heroic failure?

Not at all! Not at all! In its place, classical evidence, classically collected, is the best insurance we can buy against repeating the radical
mastectomy mistake. It's essential.

But that won't get us where we need to go—where we *can* go—if we
want better health care as a system, all together, trapped in complexities.
My friends, the world you are living in as you try to help health care get
better is a world of true complexity, strong social influences, tight depen-
dence on local context, a world less of proof than of navigation, less of
final conclusions than of continual learning, a world not of certainty
about the past, but of uncertain predictions and tentative plans about
the future. You are *I–Thou* explorers in an *I–It* world.

So, you suggest Rapid Response Teams, and someone shoots back,
"Where is the evidence?" You suggest moving toward a culture of patient
safety, and they ask, "What's the proof?" You suggest changes, and they
affirm the status quo until an RCT appears. *"Primum non nocere,"* they
say. "First, do no harm." When we, seeking improvement, forge ahead
with change anyway, the OXO evaluation world thinks we are anti-
intellectual and don't value evidence. If you're like me, that makes you
doubt not the skeptics, but yourself. You doubt yourself.

Wouldn't it be great if we could end that combat? We *do* need both.
We need to value and develop ways of knowing—scholarship—in both
types of world: in the *I–It* world—the one that looks hard at hard, cold
facts about radical mastectomies—and in the *I–Thou* world, where our
relationships, our contexts, our whole selves matter inescapably. If we
don't heal that rift between classical academic evaluation and the joy,
energy, and wonder of improvement, then people get caught in the
middle, people like you and that doctor, waving his hand in the air,
slowing you down when you wish with all your heart that you could
speed up.

To find the common ground, we need to agree on only one thing: that
how you should learn about something depends on *what* you are learning
about. It's *that* simple. The object of study and the best way to study it
are related. To study a linear, mechanical, tightly coupled causal relationship most efficiently, an OXO experiment may be just what the doctor

ordered. That's how, I think, most drugs, devices, and procedures ought to be studied. I am orthodox OXO when the question's about methotrexate for leukemia or beta-blockers for heart failure.

But, when it comes to social change—by which I mean changes, interventions, ideas that involve complex relationships, some of which are interpersonal, all of which are nonlinear, in social systems with important contextual influences, then we need methods fit for that purpose.

Pawson and Tilley do not leave us high or dry. They suggest a little model they call "CMO," which is shorthand for "Context + Mechanism = Outcome." "In other words," they write, "programs work (have successful 'outcomes') only in so far as they introduce the appropriate ideas and opportunities ('mechanisms') to groups in the appropriate social and cultural conditions ('contexts')." The *I–It* world and the *I–Thou* world want the same outcomes; they diverge in the importance they attach to contexts. Let's see how that plays for rapid response systems. Through the CMO lens: "Rapid response systems work (have successful 'outcomes,' like reductions in cardiac arrests outside ICUs) only in so far as they introduce the appropriate ideas and opportunities ('mechanisms') to groups in the appropriate social and cultural conditions ('contexts')." I think, "Yes." That fits. That's highly probable.

Pawson and Tilley say, "Most things have been found sometimes to work." In rapid response country, that would be: "Rapid response systems have been found sometimes to reduce cardiac arrests and mortality." Again, "Yes." Now, When? How? Why?

Why do OXO evaluation designs, alone, let you down? Pawson and Tilley say, "Experimentalists have pursued too single-mindedly the question of *whether* a program works at the expense of knowing *why* it works." The OXO experimental model's epistemology actually relies on—it depends on—*removing* information on context and details of mechanisms, so that its results are generalizable. It can't tell us how or what because it tries to remove variation from the "how" of mechanisms and the "what" of context. So, what makes the RCT so strong as a tool for learning in some settings makes it weak in others. If you are trying to learn, not *whether* rapid response works, but rather *how* or *when*, then evaluating it with randomized clinical trials is like trying to eat soup with a fork.

Try to make your marriage better with a randomized clinical trial, and you'll find out what I mean.

We need to learn better how to learn in a world of *I and Thou*, and that means we need a new level of maturity about evidence. We need to get out of these endless, demoralizing, frankly insulting debates about evidence, on the one hand, and improvement, on the other. It is a debate that drains energy, hope, and confidence at a time when we need all three, and it is time for it to stop.

Here are four ideas for change:

First, we need to broaden our methods of research. To improve health care outcomes broadly, we need research methods that can capture information on the details of mechanisms (who did exactly what, exactly how?) and on contexts (what influences, whether planned or not, affected the outcomes?). This search was what the Fall Harvest of the Campaign was about. Evaluators, clinicians, and, hardest of all, medical journals will have to recognize that the usual experimental paradigm—OXO— is not often up to that task. Remember, experimental control usually intends to blind us to exactly what we ought to want to know about the *how*.

The commitment to base our actions on evidence is one of the greatest advances in health care in the twentieth century. The improvement movement is its descendant, and we carry that banner. Now, we have the great challenge of improving our understanding of evidence itself to make sure that the science we use fits the questions we have. We need, not *less* evidence, but *more* evidence—more *powerful* evidence that drives broader outcomes in diverse settings. We need not *less* rigor, but *more* rigor, hewn by more and better tools in the evidence toolbox, so that we can learn more faster by harnessing the energy of many. RCTs were a giant step forward; it didn't come easy. Now we have a chance for another giant step, and that won't be easy, either.

My friend and colleague, Bob Lloyd, is a master at exploring the evidence toolbox. He explains it this way. The simple view is of linear cause and effect: X leads to Y. But the world of systems, the one we're exploring at the Forum, the causal systems look a lot messier.

Here is another way to think of it. The simple view is one-dimensional. Imagine a single line, going from simple dynamics at one end to complex ones at the other, from *I–It* to *I–Thou*, from neat to messy. The simple view is that scientific rigor, discipline in evaluation, runs along the same line—from rigorous to sloppy, hard-headed to soft, from RCT to anecdote. So, how do we learn? Answer: Strip away that complexity. Neaten things up. Neuter complexity with randomization, blinding, and objectivity. If you think that way, you try to make the mess neat so you can study it.

Here's a different view. Maybe learning and evaluation at both ends of that first line—all the way along the line—can be disciplined or sloppy, rigorous or not. That means we don't have a line, but instead we have a plane of possibility. Radical mastectomy is a rather simple case of cause and effect. The most rigorous design to find out what it does was, and still is, a randomized trial.

But, carry the RCT over to where complexity prevails, and suddenly the RCT doesn't look so good. It's actually a rather bad way to learn. What would rigor be—what are great the tools for learning—in the upper-right-hand quadrant, when the world is too messy to ignore contexts, mechanisms, and relationships—when randomization and controlled experiments make us blind to what we ought to see?

Some statistical techniques, some that developed outside medicine, in engineering, for example, do better at this—methods like statistical process control, time series analyses, and off-line experimental designs. So do anthropology, ethnography, and even journalism. When we want to understand contexts and mechanisms, they are not compromises; they are superior. What makes some ICUs skilled at welcoming families into their settings and makes others construct barriers? Different methods help us build different knowledge with different technical disciplines. If we are in the messy world, maybe when someone suggests a controlled trial, we should suggest a control chart for the outcome we seek. Maybe when someone calls for a statistician, we should suggest an anthropologist. And, yes, maybe, when someone asks for a lot of numbers, we should gather, instead, a few stories.

The second change we need is to reconsider our attitudes toward thresholds for action. When do we wait for more knowledge? And when do we go ahead, pull the trigger, act? Formal experimental designs traditionally try to avoid one particular type of error like the plague: rejecting the null hypothesis when it is true. In simple words, they're designed to keep us from saying, "It works," when it actually *doesn't* work. That's prudent when the threat of that kind of error is great, and when the status quo warrants some confidence. That's how we usually interpret *Primum non nocere*: Don't change the status quo unless you're sure.

In health care, the status quo isn't very attractive; it's ugly. So, do we actually *want* to give the status quo such a leg up? What about, maybe, "*Primum*, don't just stand there?" "When you are doing harm, find a way to stop it." Systems that humans—not nature—have designed require human action if they are to improve.

Now there are both smart ways to do that and silly ways. Let's be smart. In trying changes to try to reduce damage from the status quo, keep your eyes wide open while you do that. "Plan-Do-Study-Act," PDSA. In their *New England Journal of Medicine* editorial criticizing some improvement efforts, Auerbach and colleagues oppose "proceeding largely on the basis of urgency rather than evidence." That's a false choice. There's a third way, and it is often a better way: proceed urgently to test promising changes, and, as you do that, gather evidence to guide further choices and broader implementation. That way, we can learn much faster than if we wait for truth to emerge only from formal research processes conducted by only a few among us. Make changes and learn from them; PDSA; that's science, too.

Improvement, properly done, *is* research and learning. And, widespread improvement is widespread research. Think of it. Local knowledge is now growing every day in thousands of settings as hundreds of thousands of clinicians, managers, and others learn—people on the very same quest that Paul Goldstein was on when he asked Ann and me how he could do better, and that neonatologist was on when he told Jessica to remember the whole, and that Ed Frank was on when he put his hand on my shoulder and said to me, "Don, when you talk with a patient, you sit down." What abundance! Ignoring that learning is waste.

This way to learn isn't the same as delegating research to a small segment of the health care industry. We ought to be, not a small network of professional laboratories, but an immense network for a learning community. Formal science, housed in formal research centers, should remain pre-eminent in supplying new ideas and technologies—hard, cold facts; but local improvement can be common, continual, disciplined, and informative to all.

And this leads to the third change: we need a different way to think about trust and bias.

Surgeons who honored radical mastectomy were biased. They believed in the logic, and they saw for decades what they hoped to see. They saw better results, even though they weren't really there. Concerns about this trickster—bias—help motivate formal experimental designs. Here is that concern in the recent words of Auerbach and colleagues: "Even when direct financial conflicts of interest do not exist, any organization that has undertaken a major campaign to improve the quality of care has little incentive to invest resources in a rigorous evaluation of the effects of its efforts." In other words, "Don't trust them."

Well, is that so? Maybe that is a sophisticated view—that the actor lacks incentives to study the effects of the actions. But, stop a minute. Try these assertions on:

"Parents have little incentive to evaluate the effects of their parenting."

"Golfers have little incentive to study the effects of their stroke."

"Armies have little incentive to study the effects of their tactics."

Do you see the tension? It is between the misleading bias of seeing what we want to see and the corrective potential of purpose and sincere curiosity to find out what, after all, is happening. None of us wants the first type of bias, but attacking it too zealously can have two very toxic effects on improvement.

First, remember that OXO approaches tend to remove most knowledge of context and mechanisms by their very design. But, hold on a minute! The richest sources of good information about contexts and mechanisms are, precisely, the actors themselves. Ken Hillman knows a ton about rapid response. He knows important details. "Why did the MET system turn out to work out so well—apparently—*there* at Site A, but not *there* at Site B?" That's a very important question. Who do you think more likely knows some good answers to that question: Ken Hillman, or a third-party evaluator with data from a blinded, randomized trial?

But many formal OXO designs forbid the researcher from asking Ken, because he is biased. "Bias" is one side of a coin with two sides. The other side is "wisdom." We cannot easily eliminate the threat of bias without sacrificing the value of wisdom. It will be far better to have research methods broad enough to harvest the observations of the people who make the changes, not just the people who study the people who make changes.

The second toxicity of a narrow view of bias is that it can demotivate people, people like you, who are trying—trying hard—to make the world better. It can make you feel misunderstood, mistrusted. You're not paranoid; you *are* mistrusted. That's because too narrow a view of bias says, whether the critic intends it or not, "I can't trust you. Outsiders must judge your work; you can't."

Changing social and sociotechnical systems is human work done by human beings. Most of these people—these improvers—you—care very deeply to do a good job. You are curious and you want to learn. With some training, disciplined self-evaluation is quite possible. We need, and we can have, professionals who know how to study the effects of their own work. That's a much more hopeful and respectful approach than just leaving evaluation to third parties, alone.

And that leads me to the fourth change in our approach to evidence. We need to reconsider mood, affect, and civility.

The basics are simple: academicians—formal scientists—and practitioners—in day-to-day care—should respect each other. That's a two-way street. Practitioners show respect when they use evidence reliably in their work, when they quickly adopt effective new care, and when they quickly stop doing things as soon as they are proven ineffective. Academicians show respect when they are curious about what practitioners know and learn.

But, I think that academic centers and doctors and nurses who value science need to go one step further. They need to reflect on how their behaviors and messages shape the mood, the self-confidence, the ambition of others. People committed to science ought to supply not just skepticism, but also hope. People committed to science ought not just to judge change, but to lead change; not just to evaluate the rest of us, but to join the rest of us.

The opportunity has never been greater for health services researchers and clinicians who value science to contribute to the improvement of health care as a whole—especially for academic medical centers. They nurture our young, they guide us in lifelong learning, they are respected as the best, and they begin the day trusted and admired. Who better than them to help the rest of us—all of us—face the realities of our problems with both honesty and confidence, with both clarity and hope, with both humility and a plan for change? Who better to tell us not just all that we do wrong, but how we can do right? Who better to say when we feel less than sure, not just, "No," "Wait," "But," and "Show me," but also, and louder, "Yes," "You can," "Try," "Learn," and always, "Thank you"? "Congratulations."

Science-minded clinical leaders and academic medical centers don't ride the brakes on improving bioscience, and they shouldn't ride the brakes on improving health care as a system. They should be pushing the accelerator. They should be less the relentless skeptics of change, and far more the scouts and coaches toward a better way.

Evidence-based medicine and its crown jewel, the randomized controlled trial, are great human achievements. It's time to build on them even further. Sound ways to find sound answers in the quest for improvement are many, not few, and they go beyond narrow definitions of proper methods and proper science. We desperately need new academic pioneers to follow in the footsteps of Feinstein, Mosteller, Sackett, and Cochrane— with courage equal to theirs—new pioneers who will teach us how, properly done, evaluative science in health care can better match its methods to the nature of its questions. Maybe some of these pioneers, not quite yet discovered, are in this room today.

This is urgent: to expand our vision with more inclusive, but no less disciplined, commitments to science and evidence. It is urgent because our aim is so much grander than a good trial well published. Our aim is progress against the suffering. The prize is not a properly designed study done by a few among us according to an orthodoxy that badly needs refreshment; the prize is helping, healing, caring. The knowledge of how to learn well is the property of no one method, no one clan, and no one place; and to improve well we will need to improve learning, itself. If we do it right—and we surely can do it right—learning, to paraphrase the great American poet, Walt Whitman, "is large. . . . It contains multitudes." What waste if we ignore that wealth! The wealth is here. And the lessons we need lie not just in the *it*, but also in the *thou*. "Thou." You. The energy. Many. You are thousands. *Thou*-sands. What your eyes cannot always yet see, your hearts *can*. Trust that. Enjoy the Forum.

FURTHER READING

Pawson R, Tilley N. *Realistic Evaluation*. London: Sage Publications; 1997.

Winters BD, Pham J, Pronovost PJ. Rapid response teams—walk, don't run. *JAMA*. 2006 Oct 4;296(13):1645–1647.

Chapter 7

WHAT "PATIENT-CENTERED" SHOULD MEAN: CONFESSIONS OF AN EXTREMIST

COMMENTARY

Frederick S. Southwick, MD

IS DON BERWICK an extremist for his definition of "patient-centered care"? Perhaps in 2008 he was, but in 2013, I believe the pendulum is moving away from physician-centered care toward patient-centered care. We have not fully achieved this important goal, and there remains much to be done. The Affordable Care Act and new Medicare rules (many thanks to Don Berwick) are beginning to reward a patient-centered focus. At my health system, we truly want to improve each patient's satisfaction with the care we provide. The abbreviation HCAHPS (Hospital Consumer Assessment of Healthcare Providers and Systems) comes up daily in our conversations.

As the physician administrator for a general medical floor, I spend an hour each week asking patients about their hospital experiences. Often they are positive, but on occasion a patient expresses concerns about discharge planning, the delay of a test, the hospital menu, or the noise outside the room. The head nurse, nurse clinical leader, and I take each concern very seriously, and whenever possible we intervene. Just yesterday a patient and his family expressed concerns about the plans for his care. He didn't understand them. I called the physician in charge, expressed his patient's concerns, mentioned that we are working to improve patient satisfaction on our floor, and asked for his help. I received a warm thank you for my feedback, and the physician promised to immediately return to the patient's bedside to discuss the plans for care and to modify them to meet the patient's and family's needs.

You may ask, "Is this the exception or the rule?" To answer this question, let me share my personal experience as a patient in our hospital. In August 2012, my left foot turned white. I had been suffering from what I thought was a pulled calf muscle for more than a month. The pain worsened during walking, and I wondered if I might be suffering from vascular insufficiency, but that seemed impossible. I had a normal serum cholesterol, a normal blood sugar, and I vigorously exercised nearly every day. An angiogram confirmed that all the arteries below my left knee were occluded. Following two surgical explorations, my vascular surgeons informed me that bypass surgery would not be possible. "What do you recommend?" I asked. The head surgeon replied, "You have two alternatives: live with the ischemic pain, or undergo an amputation."

I was discharged home to allow me time to decide. What kind of life would I have without my leg? The pain was sharp and unrelenting. I could only walk three to four steps without severe discomfort. I had to sleep in a chair with my foot hanging down to reduce my pain, sleeping only in ten-minute intervals. After two weeks I made my decision: I chose amputation. At my request they initially performed a below-the-knee amputation because this afforded the greatest function. However, within fourteen days the lower part of my leg became necrotic and an above-the-knee amputation was required. I am now adapting to life with one leg.

This decision was left up to me, and my surgeons provided me with the time to evaluate my choices and accept the consequences of my treatment. That is exactly the way it should be. Central to my recovery, I will always remember and be grateful for the gentle approach and deep empathy of my caregivers. So, in answer to your question, I believe that a patient-centered focus is now becoming the rule rather than the exception.

These changes are the consequence of the unrelenting efforts of leaders like Don Berwick who have been willing to be perceived as extremist. They are the adaptive leaders we require to change the way we do things. Change angers those in favor of the status quo because they are comfortable with the current state and feel a sense of loss. Change causes disequilibrium or emotional discomfort. Those who benefit from the status quo try to reduce their discomfort in one of two ways. First they may try to delay the changes. "We don't have time to make these changes." "Things are fine the way they are." "Patients don't understand what they need." Second, those in favor of the status quo will attack the leader who is encouraging change, perhaps calling him or her an extremist.

By calling himself the very name those opposed to change might have used themselves, Don Berwick neutralized their objections. His strategic wisdom, humility, and courage have allowed him to survive as an adaptive leader. He has set an example for all those who want to and should lead change. We need to support, encourage, and protect adaptive leaders like Don Berwick. Our patients are counting on it!

FURTHER READING

Heifetz RA, Grashow A, Linsky M. *The Practice of Adaptive Leadership: Tools and Tactics for Changing Your Organization and the World*. Boston: Harvard Business Press; 2009.
Southwick FS. *Critically Ill: A 5-Point Plan to Cure Healthcare Delivery*. Carlsbad, CA: No Limits Publishing Group; 2012.

WHAT "PATIENT-CENTERED" SHOULD MEAN: CONFESSIONS OF AN EXTREMIST

KIMBALL LECTURE, AMERICAN
BOARD OF INTERNAL MEDICINE (ABIM)
FOUNDATION SUMMER FORUM
YOUNTVILLE, CALIFORNIA, JULY 27, 2008

THREE YEARS AGO, a close friend began having chest pains. She headed for a cardiac catheterization, and she asked me to go with her. As I stood next to her gurney in the pre-procedure room, she said, "I would feel so much better if you were with me in the cath lab." I agreed.

The nurse didn't agree. "Do you want to be there as a friend or as a doctor?" she asked.

"I guess both," I replied. "I *am* both."

She said, "It's not possible. We have a policy against that."

The cardiologist showed up a few minutes later. "I understand you want to have your friend in the procedure room," she said. "Why?"

Note: This speech was published subsequently, by *Health Affairs*, as "What 'Patient-Centered' Should Mean: Confessions of an Extremist." (Berwick DM. What "patient-centered" should mean: Confessions of an extremist. *Health Affairs*. 2009 Jul–Aug;28(4):w555–w565. Archived and available at http://content.healthaffairs.org/content/28/4/w555.abstract)

My friend said, "Because I'd feel so much more comfortable, and, later on, he can explain things to me if I have questions."

"I'm sorry," said the cardiologist, "I am just not comfortable with that. We don't do that here. It doesn't work."

I asked, "Have you ever tried it?"

She said, "No."

"Then how do you know it doesn't work?" I asked.

"It's just not possible," she answered. "I am sorry if that upsets you."

Moments later, my friend was wheeled away, shaking in fear and sobbing.

My question is this: What's wrong with that picture?

Most doctors and nurses, I think, would answer that what is wrong with that picture is that my friend and I were being unreasonable.

I disagree. I find a lot wrong with that picture, but unreasonable expectations aren't on my list. What is wrong in my opinion is that the system exerted its power over reason, respect, and even logic in order to serve its own needs, not the patient's. What is wrong, in my opinion, was that the system used a form of violence and tolerance for untruth, and— worse for a profession dedicated to healing—did needless harm.

It was violent because it forcibly separated an adult from a loved companion. It was untrue, because it appealed to nonexistent rules, and because it stated opinion as fact. It did harm because it increased fear when it could have assuaged fear with a single word: "Yes."

In 1998, the Institute of Medicine [IOM] established the program on Quality of Care in America. I served on the first, major IOM Committee on that topic, the Committee on the Quality of Health Care in America, and I chaired one of its two subcommittees—the one called informally the "chassis subcommittee," because our job was to suggest new designs for care. That term dated to the predecessor IOM activity, the National Roundtable on Health Care Quality, one of whose members, David Lawrence, famously said, "The problem is that the chassis is broken."

The roundtable published a landmark article in the *Journal of the American Medical Association* in 1998. It labeled the quality problems as a trio—"overuse, underuse, and misuse"—and proffered this definition of quality: "The degree to which health services for individuals and populations increase the likelihood of desired health outcomes and are consistent with current professional knowledge."

In the summer of 2000, at the Woods Hole Center of the National Academy of Sciences, the IOM Committee on the Quality of Health Care in America, and its two subcommittees held what I think was the turning point meeting of that IOM process. My subcommittee knew that no proposed redesign could be a good one without a clear definition of what should be improved: the aims of health care itself. Reducing overuse, underuse, and misuse was a good start, we felt, but the list felt incomplete. It was too technical.

In an hour, we had on a flip chart page a new framing of aims. The initial draft read, "Safety, effectiveness, patient control, promptness, efficiency, and equity." "Promptness" became "timeliness"—no problem there.

The sticking point was the third entry on the list of aims for improvement: "patient control." Our group was friendly, but it was tense as members sorted themselves into camps along a line that ran, more or less, from radical consumerism (as in, "The customer is always right") to classic professionalism (as in, "Patients make decisions that are not in their best interests," and "Does that mean that anyone who asks for a CT scan gets one?"). We thought about compromise words: *partnership*, *sharing*, *respect for patients*, and more. We settled, in an uneasy peace, on "patient-centeredness" as the aim.

The disagreement surfaced again later that same day around what became the "Ten Simple Rules" for redesign—the guiding principles of how the health care system should operate to achieve the six aims for improvement. Rule number three, drafted by the radicals, started out as "Patients have all the control." But, some argued that patients' demands would be unreasonable or unwise. Others cited patients who would choose to turn all the decisions over to their doctors, rather than keep control. Rule number three ended up as "The patient is the source of control." The third of the six aims, "patient-centeredness," and the third of the ten design rules, "The patient is the source of control," found themselves in those forms in the great chartering document, *Crossing the Quality Chasm*.

There is a big difference between the 1997 roundtable focus on overuse, underuse, and misuse as bounding the problem of health care quality, and the six aims and ten rules of the *Chasm* report. The difference turns on the third aim and the third rule, which, taken as strongly as I would have them taken, are potentially revolutionary. I think they can and should redefine professionalism itself.

The sociologist, Eliot Freidson, in his classic study of health care, *Profession of Medicine*, defines a profession as a work group that reserves to itself the authority to judge the quality of its own work. Freidson says that society cedes this authority to a profession because of three beliefs: (a) altruism—that professionals will work in the best interests of those they serve, rather than their own interests, (b) expertise—that professionals are in command of a special body of technical knowledge not readily accessible to nonprofessionals, and (c) self-regulation—that professionals will police each other.

Freidson's definition of a profession contradicts the usual assumption of consumer-oriented production, in which the customer, not the producer, has the authority, exercised by marketplace choices, to judge quality. In Freidson's world of professions, excellence is in the eye of the professional. In the more normal world of products and services, excellence is in the eye of the customer.

The latter is not a moral position; it is a pragmatic one. The business theory under modern quality strategies is that producers who meet consumers' needs, as judged by consumers, will thrive, and those who do not will wither.

The IOM Committee found itself uncomfortably torn between Freidson's form of professionalism—"Trust us; we know best what will help you; it's for your own protection"—and the consumerist view of quality—"Let us know what you need and want, and that is what we will offer." The words, "patient-centeredness" and "the patient as the source of control," are verbal analgesics, but they mask real pain.

If the technocratic definition of quality canonized by the roundtable holds, then only two of the six IOM aims are primary, and patient-centeredness is not one of them. The only two that stand on their own are safety ("avoiding misuse"—that is, doing no harm from care) and effectiveness ("avoiding overuse and underuse"—that is, grounding care in evidence). The other four aims—patient-centeredness, timeliness, efficiency, and equity—have valence only because and to the extent that they help determine safety, effectiveness, and health.

A consumerist view of quality takes each of the six IOM aims on its own merits, without forcing connection to the others, just as in judging the quality of an automobile, we can independently assess safety, comfort, reliability, gas mileage, beauty, and driving fun as separate characteristics. They may be unequal in importance, but the merit of each does *not* depend on its influence on another.

In the consumerist view, the current IOM definition of quality is defective. It is a professionally dominated view of excellence. It subordinates by implication the four lesser IOM aims to the technical triad of overuse, underuse, and misuse.

The organization that I lead, the Institute for Healthcare Improvement, regularly uses a set of "system-level measures" or "whole-system measures" of quality to characterize performance. One of these derives from our project ten years ago on the Idealized Design of the Clinical Office Practice. For that project, I personally drafted this as an overarching aim for an ideal practice: that its patients would say of it, "They give me exactly the help I need and want, exactly when I need and want it."

Note that the IHI question explicitly and uncomfortably stresses the view of care through the patients' eyes, especially with the words *need and want*, rather than *need* only. That word, *want*, is the tough word.

Along the range between the professionally dominant view of quality of health care and the consumerist view, I plant my stake far from Freidson's definition. I think it is wrong for the profession of medicine, or the profession of nursing, or any other health care profession, for that matter, to "reserve to itself the authority to judge the quality of its work." I don't like compromise words like *partnership*. I think that we—patients, families, clinicians, and the health care system as a whole—would all be far better off if we behaved with patients and families not as hosts in the care system, but as guests in their lives. And, I suggest that we should without equivocation elevate patient-centeredness to the status of a primary quality dimension all its own, and honor it not because—not *only* because—it contributes to safety and effectiveness of care.

Most researchers who have studied patient-centeredness systematically, actually, have found that it does often have a positive relationship to classical health status outcomes. This is in part because patients and families can bring useful knowledge to care if they are invited to do so.

Golomb and others, for example, found that patients on statin drugs were far more likely than doctors to initiate discussions of symptoms possibly related to the drugs ($p < 10^{-8}$). Annette O'Connor's systematic review found a 23 percent reduction of surgical interventions among patients using shared decision-making technologies, with better functional status and satisfaction. Apparently, informed patients know best what will help them. It also seems that self-esteem, authentic dialogue, choice, and learning through knowledge themselves can potentiate allopathic effects.

Three useful maxims help me grasp patient-centeredness better:

- "The needs of the patient come first,"
- "Nothing about me without me," and
- "Every patient is the only patient."

The first of these—"The needs of the patient come first"—is a pervasive slogan at Mayo Clinic. They refer often to the words of Dr. William J. Mayo: "The best interest of the patient is the only interest to be considered."

I first heard the second phrase, "Nothing about me without me," from Dr. Diane Plamping, a UK health care organizational sociologist. It calls for levels of transparency and participation uncharacteristic of most health care systems.

I first saw the third phrase, "Every patient is the only patient," at the entryway to the Harvard Community Health Plan Hospital at Parker Hill in Boston, placed there by its CEO, Arthur Berarducci. It has since signified to me the attitude of "guest" in the patient's life and an intent to customize care to the level of the individual.

As I stood in the pre-catheterization room, watching my friend be rolled away, crying, on her gurney, none of those three ideas was in evidence. The needs of the patient did not come first—the habits and rules of the doctors and nurses did. Many things were going on about her without her; the alleged rules were neither negotiated in advance nor open for discussion. And she was not "the only patient"; she was anonymous, a member of a class, and her unique needs, wants, and reasons had no voice at all in the face of blunt, deaf standard practices.

My proposed definition of "patient-centered care" is this:

> The experience (to the extent the informed, individual patient desires it) of transparency, individualization, recognition, respect, dignity, and choice in all matters, without exception, related to one's person, circumstances, and relationships in health care.

In most circumstances, people would, and should be able to, include the experience of family and loved ones of their choosing, so our actual topic should be "patient- and family-centered care."

In this view, a patient- and family-centered health care system would be radically and uncomfortably different from most today. Let me suggest a few examples:

- Hospitals would have no restrictions on visiting—no restrictions of place or time or person, except restrictions chosen by and under the control of each individual patient.
- Patients would determine what food they eat and what clothes they wear in hospitals.
- Patients and family members would participate in rounds.

- Patients and families would participate in the design of health care processes and services.

- Medical records would belong to patients. Clinicians, rather than patients, would need to have permission to gain access to them.

- Shared decision-making technologies would be used universally.

- Operating room schedules would conform to ideal queuing theory designs, not to the convenience of clinicians.

- Patients physically capable of self-care would, in all situations, have the option to do it.

This form of truly patient-centered design, which I freely admit to be extremist, will alarm a lot of health care professionals. Let me anticipate three objections, and offer some prophylactic rebuttal.

First, leaving choice ultimately up to the patient and family means that evidence-based medicine may sometimes take a back seat. On the whole, I prefer that we take the risk of overuse along with the burden of giving real meaning to the phrase "a fully informed patient." If, over time, a pattern emerges of scientifically unwise or unsubstantiated choices—like lots and lots of patients' choosing scientifically needless MRIs—then we should seek to improve our messages, instructions, educational processes, and dialogue to understand and seek to remedy the mismatch. For the same reason, we ought to abandon the word *noncompliance* when it comes to medication use. When patients fail to abide by our advice or the technical evidence, they are telling us something that we need to hear and learn from.

I can, by the way, imagine just as easily as my critics can a patient request so crazy that it is time to say "No." But my wife, a lawyer, told me long ago the aphorism in her field: "Hard cases make bad law." So it is in medicine: "Exceptional cases make bad rules." You do not successfully rebut my plea for extreme patient-centeredness by telling me that, on rare occasions, we ought to say "No." I say, "Your 'rare occasions' make for very bad rules for the usual occasions."

A second objection emphasizes the duty of the professional as steward of social resources. Is patient-centeredness of the type I envision socially responsible? No one can yet know the answer to that question. Pandora's box may be empty. O'Connor and colleagues' summary of shared decision making for surgery cuts the other way—more sharing, less invasive care; and Fisher and Wennberg's work suggests that supply drives demand, not the other way around.

A third objection concerns the needs and wants not just of the patient, but of the clinician, too. Does patient-centeredness require of the doctor self-denial and martyrdom? I think not. I believe, rather, that the moats we dig between patients and clinicians can drain spirit from both. When, in a caring relationship, we deny to the other what we could with free hearts give, we both suffer from the denial; one loses the help, the other loses the joy of helping. Among the most destructive forms of denial is the message: "You should not want that." Even more destructive is the habit of phrasing our choices as external rules. If we say, "We cannot do that," when we darn well could, we're lying.

In a remarkable essay, "A New Professional: The Aims of Education Revisited," Parker Palmer argues against definitions of professionalism that separate human beings from their own feelings and hearts. He writes, in part:

> The education of the new professional will reverse the academic notion that we must suppress our emotions in order to become technicians. . . . We will not teach future professionals emotional distancing as a strategy for personal survival. We will teach them instead how to stay close to emotions that can generate energy for institutional change, which might help *everyone* survive.

Palmer is arguing for a reconnection of the feelings of health care professionals with their work, and he believes that violence is done when that connection is sundered by institutional norms and training. Threats to the health of the professions come far more from denying our basic instincts to help than from embracing them.

Let me suggest a few design constraints on the health care system that we need and want. Let me urge the leadership of the professions—all of you—those to whom has been reserved the right to judge the quality of their own work—to give up that power.

First, affirm patient- and family-centered care as a dimension of quality in its own right, and not just through its effect on health status and outcomes, technically defined. A simple way to begin in an office practice is to ask the following question at the end of most encounters: "Is there anything at all that could have gone better today from your point of view in the care you experienced?" For quantitative ratings, ask patients to rate disagreement to agreement on a one-to-five scale with the assertion: "They gave me all the care I needed and wanted, exactly when and how I needed and wanted it." Seek fives and study the low raters.

Second, give patients and families control over decisions about care in all its aspects. Take over control only rarely and with permission freely granted.

Third, extend transparency to all aspects of care, including science, costs, outcomes, processes, errors, and injuries. Apologize when things go wrong.

Fourth, make individualized care a design target. This means creating flexible systems that can adapt, on the spot, to the individual needs and circumstances of individual patients.

Fifth, train all young professionals in these as norms of professionalism. Parker Palmer's advice to help students find and have confidence in their own emotional intelligence is key to this, as are skills in mindfulness, inquiry, and dialogue.

I freely admit to extremism in my opinion of what patient-centered care ought to mean. I find the extremism in a specific location: my own heart. I fear to become a patient. Part of that fear comes from what I know about patient safety. But, the honest truth is that, for me, the errors and unreliability are not the main reasons I am afraid.

What chills my bones is indignity. It is the loss of influence on what happens to me. It is the image of myself in a hospital gown, homogenized, anonymous, powerless, no longer myself. It is the sound of a young nurse calling me, "Donald," which is a name I never use—it's "Don," or, for her, "Dr. Berwick." It is the voice of the doctor saying, "We think" instead of, "I think," and thereby placing that small verbal wedge between himself as a person and myself as a person. It is the clerk who tells my wife or my son to leave my room, or me to leave theirs, without asking if we want to be apart. Last month, a close friend called a clinic for her mammogram report, and was told, "You have to come here; we don't give that information out on the telephone." She said, "It's okay, you can tell me." They said, "No, we can't do that." Of course, they *can* do that. They *choose* not to do that; and their choice trumps hers, period. That's what scares me. It scares me to be made helpless before my time, to be made ignorant when I want to know, to be made to sit when I wish to stand, or to be alone when I need to hold my wife's hand, or to eat what I do not wish to eat, or to be named what I do not wish to be named, or to be told when I wish to be asked, or to be awoken when I wish to sleep.

Call it patient-centeredness if you choose, but, I suggest to you, this is the core: it is that property of care that welcomes me to assert my humanity and my individuality and my uniqueness. If we be healers, then I suggest that that is not a route to the point; it is the point.

FURTHER READING

Chassin MR, Galvin RW, National Roundtable on Health Care Quality. The urgent need to improve health care quality: Institute of Medicine National Roundtable on Health Care Quality. *JAMA*. 1998;280(11): 1000–1005.

Committee on Quality of Health Care in America, Institute of Medicine. *Crossing The Quality Chasm: A New Health System for the 21st Century*. Washington, DC: National Academies Press; 2001.

Conway J, Johnson B, Edgman-Levitan S, Schlucter J, Ford D, Sodomka P, Simmons L. *Partnering With Patients and Families to Design a Patient- and Family-Centered Health Care System: A Roadmap for the Future. A Work in Progress*. Institute for Family-Centered Care and Institute for Healthcare Improvement; 2006. http://www.ihi.org/knowledge/Pages/Publications/PartneringwithPatientsandFamilies.aspx.

Freidson E. *Profession of Medicine: A Study of the Sociology of Applied Knowledge*. New York: Dodd Mead; 1970.

Golomb BA, McGraw JJ, Evans MA, Dimsdale JE. Physician response to patient reports of adverse drug effects: Implications for patient-targeted adverse effect surveillance. *Drug Saf*. 2007;30(8):669–675.

Johnson B, Abraham M, Conway J, Simmons L, Edgman-Levitan S, Sodomka P, Schlucter J, Ford D. *Partnering with Patients and Families to Design a Patient and Family-Centered Health Care System: Recommendations and Promising Practices*. Bethesda, MD: Institute for Family-Centered Care; 2008. http://www.ihi.org/knowledge/Pages/Publications/Partneringwith PatientsandFamiliesRecommendationsPromisingPractices.aspx.

O'Connor AM, Stacey D, Llewellyn-Thomas H, et al. Patient decision aids for balancing the benefits and harms of health care options. Institute for Healthcare Improvement Web site. May 2004. http://www.ihi.org /knowledge/Pages/Publications/PatientDecisionAidsforBalancing BenefitsHarmsofHealthCareOptions.aspx.

Palmer PJ. A new professional: The aims of education revisited. *Change*. 2007 Nov–Dec:5–12.

Chapter 8

TENSE

COMMENTARY

Jessica Berwick, MD, MPH

THE ESSAY YOU *are about to read contains flying elephants.*

Long before Harry Potter was a household name, my father introduced me to another Hermione, and her flying elephant, Spaghetti. Together these two went on magnificent adventures as my father gleefully imagined Hermione climbing onto Spaghetti's back, and the graceful elephant soaring up into the air.

At that time, my father was also imagining the Institute for Healthcare Improvement (IHI) into being. Twenty years later, in 2008, my father delivered this speech at IHI's National Forum. I was then in my third year of medical school, in the thick of clinical rotations: watching in awe my first thoracic surgery, witnessing my first cesarean section, observing a mentor discuss end-of-life care with an elderly man.

As I write this in 2013, I am in my third year of residency, approaching the end of my formal training in internal medicine and primary care. In the intervening years American health care has been transformed. The administration of President Barack Obama passed the Affordable Care Act (ACA), which begins to enshrine in law the principles of accessible, patient-centered, safe health care. Nearly every resident of the Commonwealth of Massachusetts, where I practice, has the security of health insurance.

My residency has spanned the latest revolution in American health care. A century ago we had few truly effective therapies. Six decades ago therapies were limited to antibiotics and a handful of basic chemotherapies. The second half of the twentieth century saw an explosion in diagnostic tools, medications, and advanced technologies, including genomics.

Only recently have we begun to ask ourselves how, and if, these myriad advances can serve the goal of health at the individual or population level. With so many more strategies for care, we are beginning to acknowledge that the gap between the patient and her health will not be closed by drug development alone. We must define health more broadly.

In "Tense," my father writes letters to me from two different futures; one is a tale of compromise and disappointment, the second a vision of success. In the first letter, frustration, disappointment, and mediocrity have prevailed in American health care. The patient comes second, or third, or maybe even last.

In the second letter, we—health care providers, administrators, policy makers—succeed in making health care safer and more equitable, centered on healing rather than rules, constraints, and perverse incentives. In the second letter, we are proud of our system and our policies, and of the impact we have on people's health and lives. The elephant takes flight.

Recently, an elderly gentleman on my service wanted to have dinner at a nearby restaurant with a beloved nephew who was visiting from overseas. We were treating him for heart failure and pneumonia; he was receiving intravenous antibiotics and intermittently requiring oxygen to maintain adequate oxygen saturation. He was connected to a continuous cardiac monitor. He understood that he would be at some risk while he was unmonitored, but he had had no major events in the preceding three days. He said, "Please. I cannot possibly explain how much this means to me." But he deferred to us, his doctors—he would not go without our permission.

A decade ago, few doctors would have countenanced such a grave deviation from the imperatives of care. (Elephants do not fly.) But a sea change is underway; my colleagues and I put our heads together and found a way to reconcile those imperatives with the prerogatives of health. The gentleman enjoyed dinner with his family, returning with healthy color in his face and joy in his eyes.

I have glimpsed both futures my father imagines in "Tense." Despite the best intentions, the demands of care can cause real medical harm. With shame and a heavy heart, I have ordered physical restraints for elderly delirious patients because there was no one available to sit at their bedsides to keep them safe. Inequalities and inefficiencies abound. Then again, I see dedicated people provide extraordinary care every day. They say, "We will find a way," when it is so much easier to say, "No, we cannot." Grounded by the duty of care, they still keep their eyes on the sky, on the impossible imperatives of health.

My father's stories of Hermione and Spaghetti delighted in the thrill of the impossible. They challenged a world full of constraints and rules and showed me the power of imagination. "Tense" doesn't feature flying elephants, but there are some who would have said that zero ventilator-associated pneumonias over four years, as Claxton-Hepburn's staff achieved, is just as improbable. This and other achievements cast a new light on the other supposedly impossible improvements in care. The list is almost endless; trust me, I hear about it every time I sit down to dinner with my father. There are flying elephants everywhere.

TENSE

PLENARY ADDRESS
INSTITUTE FOR HEALTHCARE IMPROVEMENT
20TH ANNUAL NATIONAL FORUM ON QUALITY
IMPROVEMENT IN HEALTH CARE
NASHVILLE, TENNESSEE, DECEMBER 10, 2008

DON'T BE SCARED, but you're being watched—carefully watched. The Future is watching.

Actually, the Future's here, in the room. The students—the health professions students—two hundred of them, are here.

Come sit around the fire. We'll sing songs about the past. We'll embrace the present and imagine the future.

Act One: The Past

This is the 20th National Forum. Twenty years ago was 1988—ancient history—the year when the Dow Jones Industrial Average crashed; it fell 6.5 percent to 1911.

In 1988, my kids were very young: Ben was twelve; Dan, ten; Jessica, seven; and Becca was two. We hiked all the time. I carried Becca on my back that year; the rest of the kids walked. This was a tough time for kid number three: Jessica. Her life was just getting revved up when Becca came along. "What's this?," she asked. "Wasn't I enough?" She thought things were just hunky dory with three kids. A newcomer wasn't all that interesting.

Neither was IHI in 1988. In 1988, in fact, IHI didn't even exist yet. But ancestors like Blan Godfrey, Paul Batalden, Penny Carver, Jim Bakken, and Dave Gustafson were already working together on projects

140

that would turn into the IHI in 1991, thanks to a grant from The John A. Hartford Foundation. One of those projects was a National Forum. The first Forum had about three hundred people. They heard reports from twenty-one teams in the National Demonstration Project on Quality Improvement in Health Care, reports from total strangers like Maureen Bisognano, CEO of Massachusetts Respiratory Hospital, and Jim Reinertsen, CEO of Park Nicollet. They're now ancestors, too. They're very old.

When we started IHI, we didn't imagine what would happen. We were way below the radar. Only weird people enrolled; in general, people thought, health care was hunky dory. The Institute of Medicine [IOM] reports, *To Err Is Human* and *Crossing the Quality Chasm*, were twelve years away.

We would have had to be crazy to predict what happened in the next twenty years. In those two decades, hundreds of people created ideas and improvements that have circled the planet. For example, the Model for Improvement came from Tom Nolan, Lloyd Provost, and their colleagues in Associates in Process Improvement. I have seen the Model for Improvement posted in the hallways of Mayo Clinic, in the headquarters of the British National Health Service, and in a one-room clinic in Kasungu, Malawi.

"Bundles," like the Ventilator Bundle and Central Line Bundle, came from Roger Resar, Carol Haraden, John Whittington, Fran Griffin, Andrea Kabcenell, and others in IHI's Research and Development Team. Nowadays, you'll hear the term "bundle" all over the world to discuss process reliability.

Sir Brian Jarman, an IHI Senior Fellow, brought us hospital standardized mortality ratio measurement—HSMR—which some entire nations now use to measure hospital performance.

IHI's Breakthrough Series—collaborative improvement projects—arrived in 1995. People adapted and expanded the Breakthrough Series model in the UK, Scandinavia, Australia, and dozens of other nations. In the United States, Ed Wagner adapted the model. So did SSM, the Veterans Health Administration, HRSA's Bureau of Primary Care, Michigan's Keystone Project, and many more.

IHI's Pursuing Perfection project, with Robert Wood Johnson Foundation support, aimed for system-level change in pioneering places like Cincinnati Children's Hospital, McLeod Medical Center, Hackensack University Hospital, and Health Partners. It also birthed IHI's work on system-level metrics—what we call the "big dots." IHI's IMPACT network took these and ran with them.

Paul Batalden, Frank Davidoff, David Stevens, and others authored new criteria for publication, the SQUIRE Guidelines—"standards for quality improvement reporting and evaluation."

And then there are IHI's Campaigns—the 100,000 Lives Campaign and the 5 Million Lives Campaign, which climaxes at this National Forum. Generous donors supported IHI's Campaign team, who have been helping over four thousand American hospitals improve patient safety.

The IHI Campaigns have changed the landscape of health care improvement forever, and globally. There are sister campaigns in a dozen countries. But, the most moving harvest of the Campaign isn't in the numbers; it's in the local details—the stories.

Here's a story from Claxton-Hepburn Hospital in Ogdensburg, New York. Jennifer Shaver, who manages respiratory services there, told us that they were about to reach a milestone: four years running without one single case of ventilator-associated pneumonia. Four years!

Breakthroughs like these are now countless. Ed Coffey from Henry Ford Health System gave me this remarkable report of five successive quarters without a single suicide among an extremely high-risk group of chronically ill adults.

We see hospitals at the forefront of the change we need, like Bellin Health in Green Bay, Wisconsin—steadily declining HSMRs, extraordinary patient satisfaction levels, and Medicare costs 25 percent lower than others in their region, which is one of the lowest regions in the country.

Perinatal injuries plummet at Elliot Hospital. Costs fall at Care-Oregon. Malpractice costs dive at the Medical College of Georgia. Sepsis mortality rates approach zero at Baptist Memorial. Heart attack death rates fall by two-thirds at Doylestown. Diabetes care approaches perfection at CareSouth Carolina. Standardized mortality rates down by nearly 50 percent at Owensboro.

I could spend this whole hour telling you about place after place, process after process, that are fundamentally better at what they do than when we all started back in 1988.

I wanted to be able to tell you today the rolled-up national impact of the 5 Million Lives Campaign. I can't. Measuring harm at large scale turns out to be a lot harder than I had hoped. The Agency for Healthcare Research and Quality and the National Quality Forum are both committed to developing global safety measures. And, at this Forum, an independent team of highly regarded health services researchers is reporting out on their evaluation of IHI's approach to global measurement of hospital-based injuries—the IHI Global Trigger Tool. Measuring the nation's rate of medical harm will be possible very soon; just not quite yet.

But, in voices like Jennifer Shaver's and Ed Coffey's, you can hear the success and the joy. I sent Jennifer a note to congratulate her hospital and she wrote, "I am printing your message. It . . . will be framed by our ICU staff [and] posted on our 'wall of fame.' . . . We are totally engaged, overwhelmingly committed, and exceptionally grateful." That's a voice we at IHI hear all over the nation, from hundreds and hundreds of hospitals. "Engaged, committed, grateful," they say. "Look at what we are trying to do." Incredibly, these lovely people thank us. Well, we thank them.

Oh, students, you would have been lucky to be part of all of that. I wish you could have been there. It's been fun.

Act Two: The Present

But, that brings me to the present: less fun. Students, it's a rough time. Look around you at the faces of your elders here. Not so happy. Stressed. Worry lines. See them?

Why are they so worried? Well, they're feeling a little helpless—a little beaten down. Partly, it's the economy, of course. A lot of these people have been saving up for retirement, and now they have a problem. So do their hospitals and clinics. They're watching the dominos fall, and they're scared that those dominos are going to hit the health care domino hard: costs rising at three times inflation colliding with layoffs, unbelievable governmental deficits, and declining real income. You have the safety of the long run to protect you; they don't.

But, there's more than that. They're confused. You see, the old social contract for professions—"Trust us, we'll clean our own house"—has frayed. Scrutiny is replacing "Trust me." Measurement follows measurement; contingency follows contingency; requirement follows requirement.

A cacophony of measurements, goals, and demands is deafening in this age of information—this age of battering information.

David Whyte, the master American poet who spoke at the IHI Forum two years ago, has a beautiful poem called "Loaves and Fishes."

> This is not
> the age of information.
>
> This is *not*
> the age of information.

Forget the news,
and the radio,
and the blurred screen.

This is the time
of loaves
and fishes.

People are hungry,
and one good word is bread
for a thousand.

Printed with permission from Many Rivers Press,
www.davidwhyte.com. David Whyte, "Loaves and Fishes,"
from *The House of Belonging*. ©1996 Many Rivers Press,
Langley, Washington.

"This is not the age of information, . . . This is the time of loaves and fishes." Just ask an elder sitting next to you if this is the time of loaves and fishes. They'll say, "No. This is the age of numbers, the age of accountability." This is the age of "toe the line," "targets," "standards," "measurement." This is the age of "feet to fire."

The fire is everywhere. Pay for performance, balanced scorecards, public reporting, hospital compare, physician compare, everybody compare. I chaired an IOM Committee a few years ago that estimated that an American hospital has to report on something like fifteen hundred different quality measures to somebody, someplace, every year—fifteen hundred facts like infection rates, and fire extinguisher locations, and beta-blocker compliance, and HCAHPS scores, and surgical mishaps, and on and on. It's hard to find even one loaf or fish in there. It's all information. It's chaos. A nurse called it "the gerbil cage," running nowhere. Using energy. Draining energy.

Now, students, you listen up. I am going to tell you something very important. You are not victims. You can make this a time of loaves and fishes. You can bake the bread and catch the fish yourself. And the old, worried people—I mean your elders—around you can do that, too.

In fact, they've done that, even though they don't always remember it. Take the IHI Campaigns. They've built a network unlike anything that ever existed before—thousands of hospitals and tens of thousands of people helping each other, learning, and celebrating. This doesn't *take* energy; it *gives* energy, if we use it right. Let's make a plan to use that energy; let's not waste it.

Here's a plan: "Make sense." When you're lost, and everything is swirling, and you lose your bearings, get your bearings. Have you ever been swimming on a rough day at the beach, and a big wave knocks you over, and, for a few seconds you are turning in the surf and you can't remember which way is up—where the sky is? And then you feel for the bottom, and your feet touch bottom, and then you find your footing, and you stand, and you remember where the sky is. That's what I mean.

IHI is trying to make sense in five areas.

1. *Hospitals*: Help make hospitals what the IOM calls for health care to be—safe, effective, patient-centered, timely, efficient, and equitable.

2. *The Continuum of Care*: Help willing systems to organize care over time and place, especially for the chronically ill. IHI's biggest project, STAAR (STate Action on Avoidable Rehospitalizations), is with The Commonwealth Fund, and it's focused on one great signal of integrated care: readmission rates.

3. *The Triple Aim*: That's our term for population-based care, care where responsible integrators take stewardship of three goals at once for defined populations: better experience of care for individuals, higher health status for the population, and reduced per capita cost: care, health, and cost. IHI's Triple Aim project now has over forty participants, and this will become, over time, the most important work we have ever done. Just watch.

4. *Developing Nations*: IHI is global. And that includes—that *especially* includes—the developing world, where a third of humanity suffers from burdens of illness and poverty developed countries have not seen since the Middle Ages. We are working with colleagues in South Africa on HIV and AIDS, in Malawi on maternal death rates, and in Ghana on deaths in children under five.

5. *Professional Development*: IHI is trying to shape a better future for learners in all health professions—to help young nurses, doctors, dentists, pharmacists, and managers become masters at helping to improve the systems in which they will work. So, we've started the IHI Open School for Health Professions. It will create a global community of thousands of students and faculty. It's already got more than sixty local Chapters and nine thousand enrolled students, and more are joining every day.

Now, all of these are important areas, but I'm going to focus on hospitals for a few minutes. Let me show you how we can make sense there—find the place to stand again in the swirling water.

Here is the way we in IHI are going to try to help you find your footing: The Map. The IHI Improvement Map. Let me explain.

Brent James, one of the clearest health care thinkers of our generation, has long argued that a hospital has a small set of mainstream workflows that account for a remarkably high percentage of what it does. One of these is labor and delivery, for example. Another is acute cardiac care.

The 5 Million Lives Campaign aimed at core workflows that affect safety—like infection control and medication management.

Think of a sport. How many workflows make up the map of great basketball? Well, shooting, passing, running, rebounding are on the map. Also, some cross-cutting stuff, like coaching, practicing, conditioning, scouting. I'd guess that we might map out basketball in about twenty flows. Get them right, connect them up, and your score changes. You might win.

Pop quiz: How many flows make up a hospital? It's a lot worse than basketball. After all, according to the IOM, a hospital today doesn't have just one score; it has fifteen hundred. That's quite a game.

How many processes does it take to get that game right? Of course, I don't know. But, I'll take a guess: about a hundred. If I actually map one hundred workflows—like infection control, and perinatal care, and acute cardiac care—you'll be able to think of lots of stuff I left out. There are over 155,000 ICD-10 Codes, and my map can't cover them all. But, I'll bet I can get a good chunk of what a hospital does on the screen by naming and mapping a hundred processes. Brent James once calculated that about 104 cover 95 percent of all care at his organization.

How hard could that be? What if we could map out, say, one hundred processes that explain 70 percent or 80 percent of what a hospital does, and then take that as our "sense-making" agenda for the task of improvement? Perfect them; perfect one hundred streams of work. Is that possible? Sure! If you're in the 5 Million Lives Campaign, you've already got a running start. You're already into at least a half-dozen must-have counties in the Improvement Map—like infection reduction, medication management, surgical reliability, cardiac care, pressure sore prevention, and governance, for example.

A master Improvement Map would have at least three types of processes: clinical processes (like cardiac care and safe surgery), infrastructural processes (like medication management), and leadership processes (like "Boards on Board" and training). There'd be maybe twenty or twenty-five super-processes, like infection control, and then four or five subprocesses—secondary drivers—for each. Voila! It's about a hundred. Brent's right. Then again, Brent's always right.

To the far right of those secondary processes—the actual hundred—is the chaos—the hundreds and hundreds—the thousands—of the micro-measures and reported things. The "non-sense." You can make sense of it, but only if you connect back to what really matters. You've got to face away from the chaos, and face toward purpose.

A great basketball team does not keep its eyes on the scoreboard; they execute the fundamental processes. That's *how* they score. You can do the same. If the master map of processes was right, and you found your route, then you wouldn't have to gaze at the scoreboard. The big picture numbers should change—on the left—and, lo and behold—lots of the little ones on the massive laundry list—the fifteen hundred—should break in the right way, too. It will be even better if the master Improvement Map—the one hundred—aligns with the priorities of other stakeholders—the Joint Commission, Leapfrog, the National Quality Forum, CMS, and so on. A smart map will make sense in all sorts of ways.

The 5 Million Lives Campaign formally ends today, but, of course, the work of total hospital improvement—filling out the Improvement Map, is not going to end. It's just starting. You have twelve locations to continue your work in—the former Campaign interventions. I'll add three more to the Map right now.

First, let's help with the financial crisis that we're reeling under. IHI is developing a "CFO Package," a set of immediate changes that can help reduce costs while improving patients' care.

Second, we're going to build on the successful infection control work of the Campaigns. We want to help hospitals reduce catheter-induced urinary tract infections (UTIs)—expensive, painful, risky, and preventable—and now on Medicare's nonreimbursement list of "no pay" events.

The third addition is especially exciting.

At last year's Forum, Atul Gawande—the brilliant writer and surgeon who also heads the World Health Organization's [WHO] Global Patient Safety Alliance project on safer surgery—told us about a new surgical checklist that WHO was going to pilot, with Atul as the principal investigator. Well, the results of that pilot are coming in, and the checklist works. If these finding are reproducible and generalizable, even partly, then this one change may have more leverage on avoidable complications in hospitals than almost any other change I've seen since IHI began.

I have an idea. Let's use IHI's 5 Million Lives Campaign network of "Nodes" that connects over four thousand hospitals in the largest such network for action in health care's history. Let's put it to work. I propose a sprint. IHI's Nodes and hundreds of participating hospitals can adopt and adapt the twelve changes in the 5 Million Lives Campaign over two years. Do you think we can make one more change in a breathtakingly shorter time? How about adopting and using the WHO Surgical Safety Checklist in at least one operating room in every Campaign hospital within the next ninety days? If we do that, the impact on surgical safety and outcomes ought to be rapid, you ought to be able to measure it locally, and it ought to be profound. If your surgical teams already use all elements of the checklist reliably, or if you have another checklist that works for you, that's terrific. If not, consider using the WHO checklist.

So, get on the Map—the Improvement Map. In the next couple of years, we want to invite you to improve your organization as a whole. We'll start with hospitals, but we'll move quickly into the whole continuum of care. We'll make space—a road on the Improvement Map—for every single one of you, no matter where you're starting, to play. Get settled, get organized, get leveraged, and get together. IHI will build the full Improvement Map. We'll propose a master, overarching agenda of processes whose improvement can lead any hospital as a whole system to totally new levels of performance. We will coordinate that agenda with the good work of the major influencers in the system, and most especially with the national priorities that the National Quality Forum is establishing. We'll reach out to you and we'll walk with you—at any speed you feel comfortable with. We'll meet you where you are. Together, we'll get a sense of direction, and we'll try to give you traction where, just now, you might feel you're spinning your wheels.

You know, we should do this even if there weren't a crisis. This is just growing up. It's taking charge. My kids, today, are grown. Ben is now thirty-two. After five years in the US Senate working for Chris Dodd, Ben is in law school now. Dan is thirty. He's the political expert who first gave us the idea for the Campaigns; he drafted the melody, and Joe McCannon made it into a symphony. He is also in school now—a joint MBA-MPA candidate. Becca is twenty-two, and she works for an environmental NGO in Boston.

Jessica, my third child—twenty-seven now—chose medicine as a career. She married Andrew Iliff, the son of British parents who live in Zimbabwe, where Andrew grew up. Jessica is a medical student at Yale; Andrew's a law student there. They're going to live in Africa—Zimbabwe, they hope—when their training is done. He'll work on human rights, and she'll work on global health.

The whole crew is growing up. I watch them in awe sometimes. What I admire most about them is that they all seem so much to want to make things better. On Election Day in 2008, every one of them was on a campaign trail somewhere—Ben in Ohio; Dan in Alabama; Jess, Andrew, and Becca in New Hampshire. They're worried, of course; but they won't agree to be victims. They'd rather make the future than predict the future. They're like you, students. They don't want to just read maps; they want to draw maps. And that brings me to the Future, watching us. . . .

Act Three: The Future

We here—all of us here at the Forum—are setting the table—preparing the world for my children, and for their children. Because of the career Jessica has chosen, we're preparing the world for her twice: once because, like all of us, she will some day be a patient, and once for her life as a doctor. For Dr. Jessica Berwick, as for the student witnesses here today at the Forum, we will create—or we will fail to create—the context that will give her a chance to do what she most wants to do with her career—to heal.

So, come with me twenty years into the future. I'll be eighty-two years old then. How old will you be when the harvest of our choices has become the platform for Jessica's life? What will we have to say for ourselves then—in 2028—at the 40th National Forum?

I don't know. I can report on the past, I can describe the present, but I'll have to write Jessica two letters about the future, not one. She can open them twenty years from now. One of these letters will be right. The other will be wrong. I do not yet know which is which.

Here's the first letter:

> Dear Jessica,
>
> I am so sorry. We stood together—thousands together—at IHI's National Forum in Nashville in 2008, the year when the Boston Red Sox and the Patriots lost, and Barack Obama won. The year of the financial crash, and the Iraq War still on. The year of uncertainty and fear, when retirement funds bled and foreclosures loomed. Health care was still untamed—medical injuries, unreliable care, patients voiceless, disparities rampant, and costs ripping into wallets and other social needs.

We tried hope. We found successes—a hospital went four years without a ventilator-associated pneumonia—and we celebrated them. Our rhetoric said that improvement was possible. It said that the new professional could thrive in a world mindful of interdependency, reliability, the sources of safety, and the power of patients. We tried to remember that transparency, which harms and insults in a suspicious world, enlightens and instructs in a world curious and learning. We tried to remember that a great leader does not command, she teaches, and, as our treasury grew imperiled, that the most valuable resource in caring is not a budget, but human spirit. We tried hope; we tried confidence; we tried change; but it was all too hard. We lost hope.

When we tried to claim health care as a human right, we were told we could not afford it. When we tried to say that racial gaps in health were intolerable, we were told that those gaps were not our fault. We tried to move the core of care from the hospital to the community, and then to home, where it belongs, but that disrupted too many plans. We tried to say that a developed nation can have good, solid health care for 9 percent of the GDP, but we were told that even 17 percent wasn't enough. We tried to say that the world's health is our health, and that a life expectancy of 42 years in South Africa is not just a South African tragedy, but an American tragedy; we were told that charity not only begins at home, but pretty much stays there. We said that we needed to change the way that health care in America is made and delivered, and we were told to get real, get pragmatic, that that was just not the American way. After all, we tried health care reform once, and it didn't work. So, we learned, or thought we learned, it *cannot* work.

We asked, "But what, then, will Jessica inherit? How will her life be?" And the answer was loud, "Grow up. Stop dreaming. It's a tough world, and a big system. Jessica will be accountable. She will be measured. If she does the right thing, she will be paid more; if she does the wrong thing, she will be paid less. We'll give Jessica incentives to do the right thing, and therefore—*because* of that—she will do the right thing."

I knew, of course, that they had not met you, Jessica. We climbed Mt. Rainier together when you were 15 years old. At 12,500 feet—2,000 below the summit—the weather began to close in. You remember. And our guide, Dave Hahn, told you the facts. "We have a choice," Dave said. "We can make the summit safely, but only if we take no more rests—no stopping. If you can do that, we'll try. But, if you need to rest, there's no shame in that. We'll call it a day, and head down now. It's your call, Jessica." And you said, "We're going up. I can do it." And you did.

They never met you, Jessica, the ones who thought that this was the age of information. The ones who called trust naïve; who called joy unrealistic; who called reform doomed, and renewal an extravagance. And so, with our eyes lowered and our fear, we shaped a world of contingency, and incentive, and compliance, and rules, and timid goals, and small, safe harbors, and concessions to mutable facts. We made choices and then called them "circumstances." We made rules, and then called them "reality." And we never made the space for different choices and better rules, and so the walls, like weather, closed in. It was every man for himself; every organization for itself; every nation for itself. And the winner was mediocrity. The winner was concession. The winner was timidity and haggling and smallness. And, in that, Jessica, even you got trapped.

Every day, Jessica, you are still as you always were, a good person with good words—food for thousands. But the potential of your spirit and ambition and hope end at your doorstep, and you feel too often alone.

I apologize, Jessica. We had a chance in 2008; but we chose wrong.

Love,
Dad

That's one letter. Here's another.

Dear Jessica,

It wasn't easy. We stood together—thousands together—at IHI's National Forum in Nashville in 2008, the year when the Boston Red Sox almost made it, and Barack Obama won. The year of the financial crash, and the Iraq War still on. The year of uncertainty and fear.

We almost lost hope. That would have been easy to do. The voices of anger and accusation were loud; the cynics were strong. We had learned to feel helpless. Measurements and surveillance multiplied, until our days became full of forms and fights and fears. We felt misunderstood, many of us, by the tough talk of those who didn't know us, and who thought that the only way to gain control was through restriction, requirement, and incentive, under glaring lights. I quaked that year, wondering what world we were shaping for you as a new, young doctor. Would that world know you? Would it invite you? Or would it simply read you its rules, ignorant of what you could create for it, wasting what you could create for it?

I knew that you did not turn around on Mt. Rainier. I knew that, given a world of encouragement, trust, coaching, and ambition, given a map, you would aim for any summit and enjoy the climb. But I also knew that a world of suspicion, restriction, and fear could just as easily make you doubt yourself and head for the safety of base camp, the summit left behind.

Luckily we made the right choices back then, in 2008. No, it wasn't luck, now that I think about it; it was courage. The weather was closing in, but we didn't turn around. We went faster. To the people who said that health care could not be a human right, we said, "We aren't *asking* if it is a human right; we are *saying* that it is. That's not a question; that's a decision." We decided, once and for all, that ours is too great a nation to allow the color of a person's skin to determine the length of a person's life. We knew that racial equality in health would require immense shifts in investments. But, we didn't run from those changes, we made them.

It dawned on us that we had been confusing the pursuit of health—our real goal—with the pursuit of care. It dawned on us that the best single measure of the success of America's investment in health ought to be the degree to which it can make health care unnecessary. It dawned on us that the best hospital bed is an empty bed, the best doctor visit is the one canceled because we don't need it anymore. We saw that our choices were wrong if they forced hospitals to celebrate high occupancy as success, rather than the production of health and function as success. Like drunks sobering, we saw the nonsense in calling inpatient days and specialist visits "productivity," the insanity in counting an input as an output.

We chose to change. It wasn't easy, Jessica. In 2008, every one of us was afraid. Our economy hadn't seen as bad a time in 60 years; we were staring into an abyss and we couldn't see the bottom. But that didn't stop us. We decided in 2008 to trade fear for renewal. In 2008, the "Triple Aim" became our aim—better experience, better health, and lower cost. And so, here is what we gave you.

We gave you a platform, Jessica, to do what comes naturally to you: to embrace everyone. To do that, we made health care in America—effective health care—a human right. That meant that government, one way or another, had a role in ensuring it, as it ensures all rights. That did not mean that government needed to own the care; that was just one of several options. But it did mean that, as a matter of public policy, no one would be left out—period.

We gave you a chance to help the poor. We met in Nashville, Jessica, on December 10, 2008, the exact 60th Anniversary of the Universal Declaration of Human Rights, which includes these words: "Everyone has the right to a standard of living adequate for the health and well-being of himself and of his family, including food, clothing, housing, and medical care and necessary social services, and the right to security in the event of unemployment, sickness, disability, widowhood, old age or other lack of livelihood in circumstances beyond his control." We decided, Jessica, to make it so. In 2008, our investment in improving global health soared.

We made it possible for you to look at patients as whole beings and therefore for them to feel whole. We freed you from fragmentation, Jessica. To do that, we decided that health care would be integrated across boundaries; that we would organize, pay for, and deliver what patients need—journeys, not fragments.

We gave meaning and memory to your work, and, to every patient, their own name. The key principle became that the core of the system is primary care, not hospitals, and that every person who wants a guide in their journey has a guide.

We reduced the waste, Jessica, that was so disrespectful of you and your patient. Our principle became that excessive care is as dangerous as care omitted; that often less care is better care. We embraced a duty: to excise overuse of ineffective, needless procedures, tests, drugs, and visits.

You were afraid you'd do harm, Jessica, so we gave you the tools to be safe. We made patient safety a primary, inalienable goal that leads right into the boardroom.

We decided that the education of young health professionals should match the social need, not fossilized traditions. Patients don't need lonely heroes, Jessica; they need stewards, as you wish to be, able to use your will and talent to climb a different mountain—not just to give care, but to improve care.

The naysayers were many, but they were wrong. They didn't recognize as choices what were choices. They didn't see that declaring previous choices to be immutable facts is the refuge of the status quo. They forgot that the best leaders reframe as possible what has been thought impossible. They forgot that saying, "It is our policy," means, exactly, "We choose this policy." And that what we choose, we can choose to change.

When we remembered that, our feet touched the ground, and our eyes found the sun, and the swirling waters seemed to calm, and we stood up. What we reaffirmed 20 years ago, Jessica, was simple, and it was exactly what *you* want: a moral compass and a good map and a sense of the right direction. And the direction is this: to heal. That is all. We are here to heal.

What we have chosen, we can choose to change. Jessica, we did change. Because of that, we proudly handed you a world better fit for you to do what you want to do—to help and heal as many people as you possibly can. "People are hungry," you know, and "one good word is bread for thousands." We baked the bread, Jessica. You're welcome. Here's one good word: joy.

Love,
Dad

In a Forum speech years ago, I mentioned a story from the Jewish Talmud. It occurred to me again last night.

There was a wise man—a sage—who people said could answer any question. A young man decided to unmask him. He would hide a small bird between his palms, and take it to the sage. He would ask him if the bird was alive or dead. If the sage said, "Dead," he would open his hands and the bird would fly. If the sage said, "Alive," he would crush the bird between his palms, and kill it.

The day came, and the young man stood before the sage, and he asked, "I have a bird hidden here. Is it alive? Or, is it dead?" "My son," the sage said, "the answer is in your hands."

Chapter 9

A TRANSATLANTIC REVIEW OF THE NHS AT SIXTY

COMMENTARY

Lord Nigel Crisp

IN THIS SPEECH, Don Berwick says he is a "romantic about the NHS" (UK National Health Service) and about its ideals, its framing, and its ambition; but he is also very realistic about its achievements and its need to grow, improve, and learn from others. His "love" hasn't blinded him to its faults. Don combines the ability to see both the ends and the means: to admire the goals and ambition of the NHS, and to set out ten suggestions for action and improvement—to be passionate, but practical.

This is a very important ability. The ancient Greek philosopher Aristotle writes about practical wisdom (*phronesis*) as the ability to understand both the ends and the means. In the *Ethica Nicomachea*, Aristotle distinguishes practical wisdom from wisdom—the knowledge of ends without understanding how to achieve them—and from mere cleverness—the ability to get things done without regard to the purpose or goal.

Practical wisdom of the sort that Don displays is in all too short a supply in health and health care. The NHS, in particular, has suffered from too many "wise" people wanting to preserve it as it has always been, without recognizing the need for change, and too many "clever" ones who want to change the way it works without regard to its ultimate purpose. Some of Don's ten suggestions address these clever people, begging them not to keep reorganizing the NHS and, above all, not to introduce market forces as the driver for provision. Other suggestions—such as the plea to train the workforce for the future, and the entreaty to "develop an integrated approach to the assessment, assurance, and improvement of quality"—focus on bringing about profound changes, but doing so in ways that are consistent with and strengthen the goals and values of the whole endeavor.

In this speech, Don is silent about what he and the Institute for Healthcare Improvement (IHI) have already contributed to the NHS. He was a powerful influence when I was chief executive of the NHS, helping us introduce quality improvement and spread good practices through the Modernisation Agency, the National Patient Safety Agency, and other routes. He was influential at the highest political level as well as at the clinical level. As I write, Don has once again been called upon by the UK government to help; this time in the aftermath of the failings at Mid Staffordshire Hospitals.

What might be different this time in the suggestions he makes for the NHS? Undoubtedly, the themes of patient focus and an integrated approach to quality will feature large, and his warnings about reorganizations, market forces, and the need to bring managers and clinicians together will all remain. However, five years is a surprisingly long time in health and health care, and other issues have grown in prominence.

There is the challenge of how to achieve quality and reduce expenditure and waste—not mentioned in those pre-credit-crunch days. So many managers, politicians, commentators, and now even clinicians are currently obsessed with this issue. There is an argument yet to be won here. There are those who still think all quality improvement costs money while others are concerned only with the costs and are willing to contemplate watering down NHS commitment to universality and equity with increased copayments, opting out, and greater limitations on provision. The practically wise route is to recognize that the two are compatible and, going further, that improvement methods actively contribute to both quality improvement and reduced waste and better value for money.

Another challenge that has grown in prominence is the need to achieve both better population health and improved individual care at the same time. These are, of course, the other parts of the Triple Aim that IHI has done so much to promote in the past few years: the aims of improving individual care and population health while reducing costs. The NHS is a natural Triple Aim organization, and Don will, no doubt, have views about how to steer it toward achieving the three aims in an integrated and effective way.

We can begin to see that nearly all the health and health care issues we are grappling with inside our own countries have a global dimension. The NHS has a part to play in promoting and sharing practice with the fast-growing regions and countries of Africa, India, Latin America, and China—many of whom are now planning their own universal health systems—and, at the same time, to learn from people who are innovating and inventing new solutions without the burden and baggage of the history and vested interests of more developed countries.

There is a new battle for Don to take on. Will universal health coverage in these countries be of a social solidarity type, as we have in Europe, or a private insurance model as in the United States?

A TRANSATLANTIC REVIEW OF THE NHS AT SIXTY

NHS LIVE
WEMBLEY, LONDON,
UNITED KINGDOM, JULY 1, 2008

LET ME BEGIN with thanks—twice. First, thanks for letting me work with you for almost fifteen years; this has been one of the most satisfying journeys of my entire career. My colleagues in the Institute for Healthcare Improvement feel the same. Second, thanks for what the NHS does as an example for health care worldwide.

If you're a cynic, you'll want to go get a cup of tea about now. I am going to annoy you, because I am not a cynic. I am romantic about the NHS; I love it. All I need to do to rediscover the romance is to look at health care in my own country.

The National Health Service is one of the truly astounding human endeavors of modern times. Just look at what you are trying to be: comprehensive, equitable, available to all, free at the point of care, and—more and more—aiming for excellence by world-class standards. And, because you have chosen to use a nation as the scale and taxation as the funding, the NHS isn't just technical—it's political. It is an arena where the tectonic plates of a society meet: technology, professionalism, macroeconomics, social diversity, and political ambition. It is a stage on which the polarizing debates of modern social theory play out: between market theorists and social planning, between enlightenment science and postmodern skeptics of science, between utilitarianism and individualism, between

158

the premise that we are all responsible for each other and the premise that we are each responsible for ourselves, between those for whom government is a source of hope and those for whom government is hopeless. But, even in these debates, you have agreed to hold in trust a commons. You are unified, movingly and most nobly, by your nation's promise to make good on an idea: the idea that health care is a human right. The NHS is a bridge—a towering bridge—between the rhetoric of justice and the fact of justice.

No one in their right mind would expect that to be easy. No one should wonder that, as the NHS celebrates its sixtieth birthday this week—an age at which humans recognize maturity, it seems still immature, adolescent, still searching.

You could have chosen an easier route. My nation did. It's easier in the United States because we do not promise health care as human right. Most of my countrymen think that's unrealistic. In America, they ask, "Who would assure such a right?" Here, you answer, "We do, through our government." In America, people ask, "How can health care be a human right? We can't afford it." We spend 17 percent of our gross domestic product on health care—compared with your 9 percent. And, yet we have almost 50 million Americans, one in seven, who do not have health insurance. Here, you make it harder for yourselves, because you don't make that excuse. You cap your health care budget, and you make the political and economic choices you need to make to keep affordability within reach. And, you leave no one out.

In the United States, our care is in fragments. Providers of care, whether for-profit or not-for-profit, are entrepreneurs. Each seeks to increase his share of the pie, at the expense of others. And so we don't have a rational structure of inter-related components; we have a collection of pieces—a caravan site. These disconnected, self-referential pieces cost us dearly. The entrepreneurial fragments create what the great health services researchers, Elliott Fisher and Jack Wennberg, call "supply-driven care." In America, the best predictor of cost is supply—the more we make, the more we use—hospital beds, consultancy services, procedures, diagnostic tests. Fisher and Wennberg find absolutely no relationship—none—between the supply and use, on the one hand, and the quality and outcomes of care, on the other hand. The least expensive fifth of hospital service areas in the United States have better care and better outcomes than the most expensive fifth. Here, you choose a harder path. You plan the supply; you aim a bit low; historically, you prefer slightly too little of a technology or service to much too much; and then you search for care bottlenecks, and try to relieve them.

In the United States, we favor specialty services and hospitals over primary care and community-based services. Americans are not guaranteed a medical home, as you are, and we face a serious shortage of primary care physicians. Hospitals, on the other hand, are abundant, with many communities vastly over-bedded—an invitation to supply-driven care. Coordinated care—care that keeps people from having to use hospitals—is rare; so are adequate home health care, hospice services, school-based clinics. Community social services and our mental health services are undefended, isolated, and insufficient. Public health and prevention are but stepchildren. Here, in the NHS, you have historically put primary care—general practice—where it belongs: at the forefront.

In the United States, we can hold no one accountable for our problems. Accountability is as fragmented as care itself; each separate piece tries to craft excellence, but only within its own walls. Meanwhile, patients and carers wander among the fragments. No one manages their journey, and they are too often lost, forgotten, bewildered. Here, in England, accountability for the NHS is ultimately clear. Ultimately, the buck stops in the voting booth. You place the politicians between the public served and the people serving them. That is why Tony Blair commissioned new investment and modernization in the NHS when he took office, it is why government has repeatedly modified policies in a search for traction, and it is why your new government chartered the report by Lord Darzi. Government action on the NHS is not mere restlessness or recreation; it is accountability at work through the maddening, majestic machinery of politics.

In the United States, we fund health care through hundreds of insurance companies. Any American doctor or hospital interacts with a zoo of payment streams. Administrative costs for this zoo approach 20 percent of our total health care bill, at least three times as much as in England.

In the United States, those hundreds of insurance companies have a strong interest in not selling health insurance to people who are likely to need health care. Our insurance companies try to predict who will need care, and to find ways to exclude them from coverage through underwriting and selective marketing. That increases their profits. Here, you know that that isn't just crazy; it is immoral.

So, you could have had a simpler, less ambitious plan than the NHS. You could have had the American plan. You could have been spending 17 percent of your GDP and made health care unaffordable as a human right instead of spending 9 percent and guaranteeing it as a human right.

You could have kept your system in fragments and encouraged supply-driven demand, instead of making tough choices and planning your supply. You could have made hospitals and specialists, not general practice, your mainstay. You could have obscured—obliterated—accountability, or left it to the invisible hand of the market, instead of holding your politicians ultimately accountable for getting the NHS sorted. You could have let an unaccountable system play out in the darkness of private enterprise instead, of accepting that a politically accountable system must act in the harsh and, admittedly, sometimes unfair, daylight of the press, public debate, and political campaigning. You could have a monstrous insurance industry of claims, rules, and paper pushing, instead of using your tax base to provide a single route of finance. You could have protected the wealthy and the well, instead of recognizing that sick people tend to be poorer and that poor people tend to be sicker, and that any health care funding plan that is just, equitable, civilized, and humane must—must—redistribute wealth from the richer among us to the poorer and less fortunate.

Britain, you chose well. As troubled as you may believe the NHS to be, as uncertain its future, as controversial its plans, as negative its press, as contentious its politics, as beleaguered as it sometimes feels, please lift your eyes and behold the mess—the far bigger, costlier, unfair mess—that a less ambitious nation could have chosen.

Is the NHS perfect? Far, far from it. I know that as well as anyone in this room. From front line to Whitehall, I have had the privilege to observe its performance and even to help to measure it. The large-scale facts are most recently summarized in the magisterial report by Sheila Leatherman and Kim Sutherland, sponsored by the Nuffield Trust, called *The Quest for Quality: Refining the NHS Reforms*. They find some good news. For example, after ten years of reinvestment and redesign, the NHS has more evidence-based care, lower mortality rates for major disease groups (especially cardiovascular diseases), shorter waiting times for hospital, outpatient, and cancer care, more staff and technologies available, in some places better community-based mental health care, and falling rates of hospital infection. An important, large-scale patient safety campaign has begun in England, as well as among your cousins in Wales, Scotland, and Northern Ireland. There is less progress in some areas, especially by comparison with other European systems, such as in specialty access, cancer outcomes, patient-centeredness, life expectancy, and infant mortality for socially deprived populations. In other words, in improving its quality, two facts are true: the NHS is en route, and the NHS has a lot more work ahead.

How can you do even better? I have ten suggestions.

First, put the patient at the center—at the absolute center of your system of care. Put the patient at the center for everything that you do. In its most helpful and authentic form, this rule is bold; it is subversive. It feels very risky to both professionals and managers, especially at first. It is not focus groups or surveys or token representation. It is the active presence of patients, families, and communities in the design, management, assessment, and improvement of care itself. It means customizing care literally to the level of the individual. It means asking, "How would you like this done?" It means equipping every patient for self-care as much as each wants. It means total transparency—broad daylight. It means that patients have their own medical records, and that restricted visiting hours are eliminated. It means, "Nothing about me without me." It means that we who offer health care stop acting like hosts to patients and families, and start acting like guests in their lives. For professionals made anxious by this extreme image, let me simply remind you how you probably begin every encounter when you are following your best instincts; you ask, "How can I help you?," and then you fall silent and you listen.

Second, stop restructuring. In good faith and with sound logic, the leaders of the NHS and government have sorted and resorted local, regional, and national structures into a continual parade of new aggregates and agencies. Each change made sense, but the parade doesn't make sense. It drains energy and confidence from the workforce and middle managers, who learn not to take risks but rather to hold their breaths and wait for the next change. It is, I think, time to stop. No structure in a complex management system is ever perfect. There comes a time, and the time has come, for stability, on the basis of which, paradoxically, productive change becomes easier and faster, as the good, smart, committed people of the NHS—the one million wonderful people who can carry you into the future—find the confidence to try improvements without fearing the next earthquake.

Third, strengthen the local health care systems—community care systems—as a whole. What you call "health economies" should become the core of design: the core of leadership, management, interprofessional coordination, and goals for the NHS. This should be the natural unit of action for the service, but it is as yet unrealized. The alternative, like in the United States, is to have elements—hospitals, clinics, surgeries, and so on—but not a system of care. Our patients need integrated journeys; and they need us to tend and defend those journeys. I believe that the NHS has gone too far in the past decade toward optimizing hospital care—a fragment—and has not yet optimized the processes of care for communities. You can do that. It is, I think, your destiny.

Fourth, to help strengthen local systems, reinvest in general practice and primary care. These, not hospital care, are the soul of a proper, community-oriented, health-preserving care system. General practice, not the hospital, is the jewel in the crown of the NHS. It always has been. Save it. Build it.

Fifth, please don't put your faith in market forces. It's a popular idea: that Adam Smith's invisible hand would do a better job of designing care than leaders with plans can. I do not agree. I find little evidence anywhere that market forces, bluntly used, that is, consumer choice among an array of products with competitors fighting it out, leads to the health care system you want and need. In the United States, competition has become toxic; it is a major reason for our duplicative, supply-driven, fragmented care system. Trust transparency; trust the wisdom of the informed public; but do not trust market forces to give you the system you need. I favor total transparency, strong managerial skills, and accountability for improvement. I favor expanding choices. But, I cannot believe that the individual health care consumer can enforce through choice the proper configurations of a system as massive and complex as health care. That is for leaders to do.

Sixth, avoid supply-driven care like the plague. Unfettered growth and pursuit of institutional self-interest has been the engine of low value for the US health care system. It has made it unaffordable, and hasn't helped patients at all.

Seventh, develop an integrated approach to the assessment, assurance, and improvement of quality. This is a major recommendation of Leatherman and Sutherland's report, and I totally concur. England now has many governmental and quasi-governmental organizations concerned with assessing, assuring, and improving the performance of the NHS. But they do not work well with each other. The nation lacks a consistent, agreed-upon map of roles and responsibilities that amount, in aggregate, to a coherent system of aim setting, oversight, and assistance. Leatherman and Sutherland call this an "NHS National Quality Programme," and it is one violation of my proposed rule against restructuring that I have no trouble endorsing.

Eighth, heal the divide among the professions, the managers, and the government. Since at least the mid-1980s, a rift developed that has not yet healed between the professions of medicine formally organized and the reform projects of government and the executive. I assume there is plenty of blame to go around, and that the rift grew despite the best efforts of many leaders on both sides. But, the toll has been heavy: resistance, divided leadership, demoralization, confusion, frustration, excess economic costs, and occasional technical mistakes in the design of care. The NHS and the people it serves can ill afford another decade of misunderstanding and suspicion between the professions, on the one hand, and the managers and public servants, on the other hand. It is the duty of both to set it aside.

Ninth, train your health care workforce for the future, not the past. That workforce needs to master a whole new set of skills relevant to the leadership of and citizenship in the improvement of health care as a system—patient safety, continual improvement, teamwork, measurement, and patient-centered care, to name a few. Scotland announced last week that all its health professionals in training will master safety and quality improvement as part of their qualification. Far be it for me to suggest copying Scotland, but there you have it. I am pleased that Lord Darzi's "Next Stage" report suggests such standards for the preparation of health care professionals in England.

Tenth, and finally, aim for health. I suppose your forebears could have called it the NHCS, the "National Health Care Service," but they didn't. They called it the "National Health Service." Maybe they meant it. Maybe they meant to create an enterprise whose product—whose purpose—was not care, but health. Maybe they knew then, as we surely know now, even before Sir Douglas Black and Sir Derek Wanless and Sir Michael Marmot, that great health care, technically delimited, cannot alone produce great health. Developed nations that forget that suffer the embarrassment of growing investments in health care with declining indices of health. The charismatic epidemics of SARS, mad cow, and influenza cannot hold a candle to the damage of the durable ones of obesity, violence, depression, substance abuse, and physical inactivity. Would it not be thrilling in the next decade for the NHS—the National Health Service—to live fully up to its middle name?

Those are my observations from far away—from an American fan, distant and starry-eyed about the glimpses I have had of your remarkable social project. The only sentiment that exceeds my admiration for the NHS is my hope for the NHS. I hope that you will never, never give up on what you have begun. I hope that you realize and reaffirm how badly you need, how badly the world needs, an example at scale of a health system that is universal, accessible, excellent, and free at the point of care—a health system that is, at its core, like the world we wish we had: generous, hopeful, confident, joyous, and just. Happy birthday!

Chapter 10

THE EPITAPH OF PROFESSION

COMMENTARY

Christine K. Cassel, MD

TELLING STORIES IS basic to most kinds of effective communication, and making them very personal stories adds enormously to their effectiveness. Stories stick because we can remember them better than principles or arguments and because they say as much in what is left to our imagination as in what is made explicit. Dr. Berwick is masterful at the use of stories to convey memorable and vivid messages that are vital to the humanistic core as well as the modern challenge of medicine. Think about "Escape Fire" (Berwick's plenary address at IHI's 1999 National Forum), a story of firefighters that became an iconic way to talk about patient safety, and his Yale School of Medicine commencement speech about the cruelty of not allowing loved ones to be with us when we are sick, reminding us that health professionals are the guests in the room (Chapter Twelve of this volume). His speech about Isaiah, survivor of a bone marrow transplant who succumbs to poverty, despair, and addiction, turns "noncompliance" into insight and compassion (Chapter Fifteen).

In the John Hunt Lecture, Berwick again uses a deeply personal story—his own father's—to explain the otherwise dry and theoretical notions of professionalism as they

surround the young physicians graduating from medical
school today. His father, Dr. Philip Berwick, was a saintly man
in the view of most of his patients; he took only two
vacations in the forty years that his son remembers, and he
was available to his patients 24/7. He was also "arrogant," his
son tells us, becoming angry at a patient who dared to
question him about a therapy recommendation. Today we
would extol the informed patient asking questions, as a way
of "Choosing Wisely," and we call that "shared decision
making." Berwick wants students to learn to engage with the
patient's values and spend time explaining the evidence,
the risks, and the benefits of proposed therapies. His father's
approach to professionalism was bounded in a different time,
but still grounded in principles of devotion to what is best for
the patient. Today we want the patient's values to be central
to figuring out what is best.

Scholarly interest in professionalism has increased over the
past decade, with a proliferation of articles, books, and
guidelines. Experts who study the profession of medicine
believe this is related to the threats to the notions of
autonomous professionalism that Philip Berwick embodied,
and a desire to reclaim the notion but on modern terms.
What does it mean to reclaim professionalism in 2013?
Berwick describes it well in a storytelling way in this speech—
that the more we know about prevention of errors, about
personalized medicine, and about the depersonalizing threats
of technology, the more professionalism requires us to become
managers and team members as well as healers.

For one thing, it requires letting go of the power and the
powerful word *autonomy*. No one in the modern world of
medicine is or should be autonomous. As Berwick so clearly
states, the demands, the complexity, the immensity of the
knowledge required, and, most important, the clear knowledge
of what serves patients best, all demand that interdependency,
teamwork, and effective knowledge of working within
systems are the ways to achieve the best outcomes for
patients, to reduce errors, and to minimize waste. But
developing competency in systems-based practice does not
reduce the importance of personalized approaches to each
individual patient; ideally, it should free the physician

to exercise that responsibility and find meaning in that privilege.

The humanistic and intuitive side of the physician's challenge is part of the professionalism that Berwick describes in the Hunt Lecture. Yes, there are many demands on twenty-first-century physicians in America for accountability to consumers and payers, but the really rewarding and deeply personal aspect of professionalism is the relationship with each patient and family, coping with the risks posed by both illness and treatment. Here the authority of the clinician can be deeply comforting even in the face of uncertainty. And Berwick reminds physicians that they have power to reclaim this terrain when it seems to have been grabbed by the regulators or the payers.

Educators are striving to inculcate the ideals of professionalism in medical students, but we are encountering a sobering reaction when this noble ideal is diminished to behavioral traits such as showing up on time for rounds or dressing in clean and nice-looking clothes. Medical students are smart, and they can figure out what is expected. If professionalism is reduced to timeliness and a dress code, the real lineage from Dr. Philip Berwick will have been lost. Even if it was a very different time, and even if many of his behaviors would be considered unacceptable in today's world, the fundamental commitment to the work of patient care, to understanding it as a privilege and to experiencing the joy of working for a goal beyond self-interest, is the lesson both Dr. Berwicks can teach us.

And therein lie the stories. As Don Berwick reminds us, the story is the patient's story. The most expert diagnosticians and the most revered clinicians are the ones who know the patient's story as well as being able to tell their own.

FURTHER READING

"Choosing Wisely" is an initiative of the ABIM Foundation. Learn more at: http://www.choosingwisely.org/.

THE EPITAPH OF PROFESSION

JOHN HUNT LECTURE, ROYAL COLLEGE
OF GENERAL PRACTICE
BOURNEMOUTH, ENGLAND, OCTOBER 2, 2008

AS A VERY young child growing up in a small town in rural Connecticut, I would half-awaken at some dark early morning hour, stirred by the sound of my father's car starting in the driveway. My father was a general practitioner in our town—one of only two. He was up because he would have gotten a telephone call that night from Mrs. Baron or Mr. Bishop—maybe Izzie had chest pain or Millie had a high fever. He would have dressed, rubbed the sleep from his eyes, and climbed into his car to make the house call. I would drift back to sleep, and maybe in the morning I'd hear a bit of the story—Izzie was in the hospital, Claire was in labor. Someone had been born. Someone had died. That night, my mother might bring dinner to Millie to help her out.

Once a day—once every single day for forty years—my father would drive the seventeen miles to the local hospital to make rounds on his patients, then return to his office for morning consultation hours, and afternoon hours, and, several days a week, evenings. His work, our town, our lives were one, in rhythm. My sixth grade schoolhouse window

---

Note: This speech was published subsequently, by the *British Journal of General Practice*, as "The Epitaph of Profession." (Berwick DM. The epitaph of profession. *British Journal of General Practice*. 2009 Feb 1;59(559):128–131. Archived and available at http://www.ncbi.nlm.nih.gov/pmc/articles/PMC2629825/)

overlooked the road that connected my father's office to the town center, and we would hear the whine of his engine as he accelerated recklessly along the road. His fast driving was famous in our town; he seemed to think he was immortal. My classmates would mutter as they heard his car speed by, "There goes Dr. Berwick." They never even needed to look up.

My father was not just a very good doctor—he *was* that—but he was also, in a small town, royal. He was a person of privilege. His privilege was to enter the dark and tender places of people's lives—our people. He knew secrets. He knew—we didn't—that Mary, browsing the market shelves next to us for her cereal, had miscarried again; that Nicholas, who sold us shoes, was struggling with alcohol; that Maureen, our Cub Scout leader, was quietly beside herself because Jonas was depressed and using drugs. He knew that Mrs. Kraszinski, who taught fifth grade, had lung cancer and was going to die from it, even though *she* didn't know, because they hadn't told her yet.

For me, this was romance. I loved my father, but I also loved what he did; who he was in our town. I loved the way people looked at him, trusted him, named their children Philip after him. I loved that the constable would never give him a ticket, even though my father never saw a speed limit he didn't break. I loved that he knew secrets, and that he helped.

Thank you for the gift of Fellowship in this College. Given my roots—given my father—it is impossible for me to overstate how meaningful this is to me. If I can beg your pardon, I accept this fellowship in honor of my father, Philip Berwick, from whom I received the compass for my own career. He died in 1995, at age eighty-four.

Never, for a single day as a child, did I want to be anything but a doctor. Few days as an adult have been different. Why, when you can be royal, would you want to be anything else?

I once asked my father what he liked the most about being a doctor. He didn't say, "Privilege," he said, "Mysteries . . . solving puzzles." He enjoyed the search for diagnosis, the making of sense from the clues and pieces. He knew this was important work, and he expected support for it. The hospital administrators, he assumed, served him. With his great responsibility came great authority. Sometimes arrogance came, too. I was eleven years old. At dinnertime, the telephone rang. A patient was calling. I watched my father listen, and then scowl. "I'm the doctor," he seethed. "You're not. You'll get penicillin when I say, and not a moment sooner." He slammed the phone handset down so violently that its plastic cradle shattered, sending shards into my beef stew.

The great medical sociologist, Eliot Freidson, in his masterpiece, *Profession of Medicine*, defined a profession as a work group that reserves to itself the right to judge the quality of its own work. Society, he said, cedes that right to the professional because of three assumptions: the assumption of expertise—that the professional has technical knowledge not accessible to the layperson; the assumption of altruism—that the professional will place the interests of those served above self-interest; and the assumption of self-scrutiny—that professionals will regulate each other, without the need for outside interference. My father, every day, assumed the right to judge the quality of his own work—he was a harsh judge, harshest of all to himself. My mother died of cancer when I was fifteen years old, and my father never forgave himself for not having detected it sooner—which was impossible. He shouldered fully and without complaint the obligations of technical mastery, altruism, and self-regulation. His bedside table was piled high with medical journals. He took only two vacations that I can recall.

My father was happy in his work, then. Today, I think, he might not be. Today, my father would be confused. His assumptions—the foundations of his personal mission and professional pride and joy—would be under attack. He would feel the same in the United States or in the United Kingdom. He would have a rough time.

He would ask, "Why do they doubt me so?" He would feel watched. He would not understand why. Strange words would swim around him, overheard from corridors he would not recognize, spoken by people he never met: *accountability, performance management, pay for performance, clinical guidelines, patient empowerment, the health care market, value purchasing*—words of surveillance, of suspicion. Not words of privilege; words of requirement, reward, and punishment. He would hear over and over again about systems and safety and standards. And, he would think it all to be nonsense, waste, off the point, insulting. He had trained, he would say, for a decade, up long nights and tense at the bedside, fighting off sleep to help, so that he could focus his time and skill and will and mind on the hard and noble task of solving mysteries for those who were suffering and putting their lives in his hands. I know what my father would say. He would say, "Go away. Let me do my work. Leave me alone. You are wasting my time." He would be angry. He would sound arrogant. He would once again shatter the telephone in disgust. He might say again, "I am the doctor, and you are not."

I would want, of course, to ease my father's pain. What could I say to him?

I could say this. Dad, things change. You know that. When you were born, there were no airplanes or computers. Two world wars still lay ahead. You began to be a doctor before penicillin was discovered. Things change.

Technology has changed—it has taken over in some ways. And each technology brings with it specialization. You took your own X-rays, right there, in your office. There were no CT scanners . . . no MRIs. That's over. You couldn't fit the machines into your office, even if you knew how to use them, which you do not . . . which you cannot.

Audacity has increased, and with it, hazard. You watched, helpless, as people died from failing organs that today can be replaced. All children with leukemia died—remember Eleanor? Today, they live, unless they die from what we do to them.

With the technology—to enable the audacity—come new institutions to house them. Hospitals beep and throb with devices—monitors, pumps, respirators—that demand departments and spaces you never met or saw in your time. Each institution becomes its own master—self-referential, proud, inward looking, and the care that you once housed almost in totality in your office—the knowledge you stored, almost in totality, in your mind—these have been divided and redivided into compartments named not just for diseases and organs but for phases of disease and parts of organs. Could you have imagined, Dad, that one day there would be a hospital that cares only for cancer or a surgeon who works only on knees? Journals publish ten thousand clinical trials every year. Memory fails; it's not up to the job anymore. What a harsh truth, Dad: you are not up to the job anymore—not alone.

And then, Dad, there is the money: trillions and trillions of dollars—in the United States, one-seventh of our economy. Hospital CEO salaries rise into the millions of dollars. The founder of a health care insurance company leaves with $1 billion in his pocket. The fate of entire governments rises or falls on whether or not they can keep some level of control over health care costs. Dad, you may still be royalty when you close the door and sit with a single, fearful patient. That patient, mostly, still trusts you—reveres you, but the reverence ends at the consulting room door, and, out there, outside your tiny kingdom, new dynasties rule. You have no idea what *power* means today in health care. You have no idea. You once had power. But now, you share power.

And, Dad, remember that definition of a profession—"reserving to itself the right to judge the quality of its own work"? That's over. I don't really know why. Somewhere along the way, the bond of public trust broke. Those assumptions—technical mastery, altruism, and self-regulation—they lost the high ground. The assumption of technical mastery weakened as evidence grew of tremendous, unexplained variation in the patterns of practice, evidence that came with our new data systems. You never knew that Dr. Harwich ordered X-rays three times as often as you did. Dr. Harwich didn't know either. Now, you both know, or can know, and so can the insurance company that pays you. And, frankly, so can the newspapers. Your private work space is now flooded with glaring light.

Altruism? What happened to faith in altruism when that insurance executive walked away with $1 billion? When that drug company manipulated the evidence on the toxicity of its cash-cow drug? When hospital managers and doctors fought bitterly and openly about their own prerogatives? When politicians swapped slogans instead of seeking wisdom?

Self-regulation? What about Shipman (the UK general practitioner turned murderer)? What about Bristol (the UK hospital where excess deaths after pediatric surgery were found)? When the guilds oppose transparency? Your patients, remember, are also citizens. And they are a bit fed up with corporate scandal and the greed of wealth and the untruths of politicians and the half-truths of advertising. Your work has not stayed immune to fraying confidence in the public at large, not immune to the public's fear of harm from pollutants they cannot see and that no one admits to.

The millennial generation is ascending—the generation that makes its own self its project, that assumes choices, and that always doubts power—the generation that says, "I am the customer, and you're not," and slams down the phone in anger. Your pride, which was your greatest asset in a trusting world, is now your greatest weakness in a doubting one. Consumerism is outpacing the social contract of professionalism.

Above all, Dad, this has changed: you now cannot do it all alone. The tasks of healing have simply passed the capacity of any single human mind—no matter how skilled or altruistic or self-surveillant. You—and your patients—have now become irrevocably part of something far larger than yourself, and the *craft* of care has transformed into the *machinery* of care. Science and system have swamped art and autonomy. In return for possibility—in return for miracles—you have paid a dear price. The price is that you have lost control. If you define yourself by that sense of control, then the price has been even higher: you have lost self.

Is this the epitaph of profession, itself? Honestly, my father might think so. He would focus on the losses—the dear price of complexity, hazard, institutional growth, consumerism, transparency, financial costs, and, everywhere, doubt.

But, I would want to help my father. I would so badly want him to take a deep breath and intercept his own grief. I would try to help him say this: "I am a child of the Great Depression and I am a soldier of World War II. I have gotten through changes before and survived. Maybe," he might say, "I'll take another look. There is a way through this. I know it."

How can I thrive—have pride—do with my life what I wish to do when the world has changed so much? When I can no longer thrive alone, but thrive only in interdependency? When I must ask less, "What do I do?," and more, "What am I part of?" When the light glares, and what I do is visible to others, even strangers, even when I don't want it to be visible? When my patients wish to control knowledge and choices and devices and drugs that, before, I—only—controlled? How can I thrive when the weakness of my mind—of any mind—fails in the task of knowing what I need to know in order to help? When I cannot alone ensure the safety of the patients in my charge? Where is my pride when an email has to replace a touch on the arm?

Is this the epitaph of profession, or the reconsideration of profession? In the former lies grief. In the latter, possibility.

What if we choose to change? Could we craft joy from loss, pride from revision, and excellence from invention?

Yes, we can, but not through reversion to the professionalism of the past—the professionalism of Freidson. Rescue—I think the stakes are no less than that—lies in the reinvention of professionalism in a world on new terms of engagement. The terms are these: complexity, interdependence, pervasive hazard, a changing distribution of power and control, and, borne on the back of technology, distributed, democratized capacities that my father could not ever have even imagined. Further, especially in my country, but even so in yours, the terms of engagement include a more precise and demanding sense of how health care links to the greater commons—a sense that we are stewards together, not just of health care resources, but of the limited resources, writ large, of our nations and our planet.

The new professional—the professional we need—is equipped, as my father, on the whole, was not equipped, with attitudes, skills, and knowledge like these:

- An embrace of citizenship in the greater whole that is health care, even when caring for a single patient. With respect to that whole—the system of care and caring—this means asking, not just, "What do I do?," but also, "What am I part of?"

- The skills to play that part—that membership role: cooperation, teamwork, inquiry, dialogue. These are more like the skills that make two parents great parents than those that make one artist a great artist.

- The skills less to *know* answers than to *find* answers. The romantic view—held tightly—romantically—still both by patients and physicians—that expertise means knowledge in the mind is now simply a myth. It bears no reasonable relationship to the realities of the flow and accumulation of science in medicine today—thousands of journals, tens of thousands of studies, rapidly changing clinical armaments facing rapidly evolving disease challenges. My father said, "I know." The new professional says, "I can find out."

- Embrace of the authority and autonomy of patients and families in a wholly new distribution of power and knowledge. Some say that doctors and patients should now be partners in care. Not so, I think. In my view, doctors are not their patients' partners; they are guests in their patients' lives. They are not hosts. They are not priests in a cathedral of technology. I have heard sarcastic doctors refer to the knowledgeable patient as "Internet positive," as if that were a challenge or a mistake. It isn't. It is self-efficacy beyond anything my father could have imagined.

- Willingness to trade prerogative for reliability. That's a subtle trade—surely the toughest one for my father, to be handled with caution. Overshoot, and patients lose the benefit of the poetry and art of individual expression from each caring doctor; but, undershoot, and patients play dice—gambling that this particular doctor knows that particular fact—up to date, accurate, and precise. The aim is to promise every single patient the benefit of the best possible science, and that inevitably places the autonomy of the individual physician in some jeopardy. But, the new professional must make the choice: either treat the patient—*your* patient—according to your own store of knowledge and facts, or give up total self-reliance so as to promise the patient—*your* patient—treatment according to the entire world's store of knowledge and facts. That promise—the promise of science—is a different kind of promise from the one my father made. He promised to do his best; the new professional promises to do the world's best.

I could go on, but I need not. You in the Royal College of General Practice know full well the transition of professional values, norms, expectations, and habits of which I speak. You are living through it here in the United Kingdom no less than we are in the United States. And you know better than I do the troubles of that transition—the grief, the conflict, the suspicions, and the doubts.

But, maybe you also can see the daylight. As I would counsel my father, so I counsel you and myself: this is a time of loss, I know, but it is also a time of great discovery. I cannot promise you comfort—it was a glorious time when our privilege as physicians, earned through expertise, altruism, and self-regulation, sufficed for our communities and our tasks. We need now to find the joy and pride—we *can* find the joy and pride— that lie in slightly different places—the warmth of teamwork, the excitement of the expedition together into the vast terrain of modern knowledge, the humor and vivid ambition of the millennial generation, the benefits to our patients from the miracles of technologies, with their risks tamed by humility and infinite caution.

I may sound naïve; my father surely may have thought so. But I hold to this, and I would tell him: the essentials have not changed. What mattered to my father at the core—not in the casing, but at the core—has not changed. My reverence for his mission—not for his trappings, but for his mission—has not changed. We are more bound together now, depend more on each other, are more clearly part of possibilities larger than ourselves. But, still, we are fortunate. Still, it is our privilege to enter into the dark and tender places of people's lives, where, still, trust abounds when human beings turn to us in their pain. Still, there will come the middle of the night, and, with it, we still have our duty to meet and our quiet promise to keep: to bring comfort. And, in the morning, still, there will be thanks.

Chapter 11

SQUIRREL

COMMENTARY

Diana Chapman Walsh

I FIRST LEARNED that Donald Berwick was giving spellbinding talks from David Calkins. This was a decade or more ago, when David was helping build the scientific foundation for IHI's 100,000 Lives Campaign. A physician to his core, as had been his father before him, David was passionate about IHI—what it stood for, how it worked, its successes, and its promise—for patients and for health care policy, for us all. Year after year, David would lug his computer all over the country to reunions of our Kellogg Fellowship group so he could buttonhole anyone who would listen to Berwick's latest talk.

Then, in late 2003, David was diagnosed with glioblastoma, the disease that had taken his father in his mid-fifties, too. What David really, really wanted was to live. And he did, for two-and-a-half years, beating the odds, treasuring every remaining day, and laying down memories with Chris, the son he so ached to accompany through adolescence as his father had been denied the pleasure of doing for him. It seemed to many of us closest to David in those heartbreaking months that, next to his family, it was his work at IHI that was keeping him alive.

He missed this speech, this "Squirrel" story. He would have loved this one. It had all the elements he wanted us to savor in a Berwick keynote: the lyrical variations in structure and

mood, the artful weaving of the personal with the
professional, the staccato of specific facts in counterpoise with
leisurely, vivid portraits, the precise use of the perfect word
around the bend of every sentence. No one is better than
Berwick at arriving—after twists and turns—at the sublime
and rare destination Oliver Wendell Holmes named "the
simplicity on the far side of complexity."

So this keynote has all of the virtues David admired, and
more. The willingness to take a risk? Who else would interject
a small-group exercise midway through a keynote address
in a cavernous ballroom with an audience of thousands? It
worked. We really, really remember—those of us who were
there—what we said to each other that day.

Fresh ideas? Berwick always introduces the IHI faithful to
thinkers and concepts from distant realms, not just out of the
building, but out of sight and out of mind. He stretches our
minds. To Turkey, where Elinor Ostrom's fishermen know
how to be grown-ups and conserve the resources on which
they depend. To colonial America's commons and from there
to the global macroeconomy, where the action for quality
improvement is moving, he predicts. And has it ever! To a
birch grove on a snow-covered ski trail where a red squirrel
awaits a man skate skiing along on his own imperfect knee.
And out along the horizon, to his grandson Nathaniel's
future, the future in which we all have a personal stake if
only we will still our hearts to notice what truly fills them.

So we have all that artistry, and we have Berwick's
characteristic coda, his rousing charge to rally 'round and do
even more: We've come a long way, but we see a long road
ahead. And here's a seven-point program for the coming year.
Come back a year from now and we'll review how we've
done. And then we'll pull up our socks again and craft some
more solutions.

Solutions. Creative solutions. Adumbrated so often in these
Berwick annual reviews. You can track the history of health
system reform in this series of talks. Here the Affordable Care
Act (ACA) may or may not become law and the IHI Open
School is just finishing its first year. Four years later, we are
implementing the ACA, and the Open School, a Berwick
brainchild, is a sturdy bridge to Nathaniel's future, a social

movement engaging and educating next-generation leaders (more than a quarter-million so far) to carry on the cause of health care improvement.

Tomorrow's leaders will need Berwick's stunning ability to bridge and balance tensions without collapsing them, to hold contradictions. Like those between power and love, love as the drive to sustain unity and maintain connections. "Power without love is reckless and abusive," Martin Luther King Jr. said in the last weeks of his life, "and love without power is sentimental and anemic. . . . [The] collision of immoral power with powerless morality . . . constitutes the major crisis of our time."

In the power of his words and of his work, Donald Berwick is teaching a moral leadership that is the essence of love. And so, in the end, it must come down to individuals: to David and his dream of a health care system that is fair, just, and safe; to Nathaniel and the world he deserves to inherit from us.

SQUIRREL

PLENARY ADDRESS
INSTITUTE FOR HEALTHCARE IMPROVEMENT
21ST ANNUAL NATIONAL FORUM ON QUALITY
IMPROVEMENT IN HEALTH CARE
ORLANDO, FLORIDA, DECEMBER 8, 2009

THIS IS IHI'S 21st Annual National Forum. That's a milestone. We're twenty-one years old—adults now. But, that doesn't mean we can't have a party. So, let's start by celebrating. We have a ton to celebrate.

You want safe care? Sentara Williamsburg Hospital: five continuous years without a single ventilator-associated pneumonia.

You want reliable care? Palmetto Hospital has cut standardized mortality rates in half. Henry Ford Health System has cut suicides in high-risk patients to zero for over a year.

Do you want patient-centered care? Southcentral Foundation, the Alaska Native–owned health care system in Anchorage, is revolutionizing primary care, knocking the socks off urgent care utilization and needless hospitalizations. Gundersen Lutheran in La Crosse, Wisconsin, is offering that community world-class care for people approaching the end of life at a cost 29 percent lower than the average cost of the last two years of life in the United States.

Do you hate waits and delays? Cincinnati Children's Hospital has nearly eliminated what they call failures in patient flow. Virginia Mason Medical Center cut ED diversion time by 90 percent.

Are you against waste? Denver Health has saved $33 million with Lean production projects. John Toussaint's ThedaCare Center for Health Care Value is adapting Lean production now in dozens of hospitals.

And what about equity—justice? We are seeing some of the best chronic disease care innovations in the United States in the resource-constrained setting of the Indian Health system.

Bravo! The health care quality movement is saving lives and reducing suffering for millions of people. We've still got a big job, of course: to make these exceptions the new normal. But now, more and more, we know what works.

And the youth are mobilizing. The IHI Open School for Health Professions is just one year old, and we have over fifteen thousand students and seven thousand faculty members—in medicine, nursing, dentistry, health administration, osteopathy, pharmacy, engineering, and more. They've taken over fourteen thousand online courses on safety, quality improvement, leadership; they've formed over 170 local Chapters on their campuses in 24 nations.

Another success: IHI's Improvement Map, an online resource to help hospitals organize their improvement work. I introduced the Map at last year's Forum, and now we've created a companion membership program we call "Passport" to help your front-line teams get down to work on the processes in the Map. The Map helps you prioritize; Passport helps you with projects to get it done.

My favorite success story of all this year comes from Africa: Ghana. IHI is there thanks to a grant from the Bill & Melinda Gates Foundation. We're partners with the largest health care NGO in Ghana—National Catholic Health Services, headed by its brilliant CEO, Dr. Gilbert Buckle, and with the government's Ghana Health Service. Dr. Nana Twum-Danso is the IHI lead. It's called *Project Fives Alive!*, and the name tells our purpose. We're trying to reduce deaths of kids under the age of five. Almost 10 percent of children in Ghana die before they are five, and almost every one of those deaths is preventable.

When I visited Ghana this year, we were working with twenty-five community health centers. Let me tell you about a standout: Zorko Clinic, in the Upper East Region of Northern Ghana. Zorko serves a subdistrict of sixteen thousand people, and in the fifteen months up to this October, they haven't had one single neonatal or child death—not one. Remember, that's in a region where more usually one in ten kids doesn't get to age five. Zorko has now gone six *years* without a single maternal death. I asked Nana how Zorko did it. Her answer was, "Hajia Mary Issaka—you've got to meet her." So, I did.

Hajia Mary Issaka is the nurse-midwife who had run the Zorko Clinic for the past five years. She and her staff greeted us on the porch of the clinic. A young boy smiled and brought us a bench to sit on.

I asked, "What's your secret? How do you save that many lives?"

I'm never going to forget her answer. Hajia Mary said, softly, "Respect. The most important thing is to respect the woman who is coming to us for help. When a woman comes here to Zorko, we smile at her. We thank her for honoring us. We give her zoomkoom." (Zoomkoom is a traditional, spicy porridge taken in the villages to help with childbirth.) "We offer her hot water for a bath," Mary said. "If she is dirty, we never, never say, 'You are dirty.' We say, 'It is hot and we are all sweaty. Perhaps you would enjoy a bath.'"

She said, "If we respect the people we want to serve, and if we show them that we respect them, then they will give us a chance to help them. If not, they won't. This is the secret: respect." Keep that thought—we'll come back to it.

I am celebrating something pretty special, myself: my first grandchild. Nathaniel Peter Iliff was born on July 13, 2009. His parents are Jessica, my third child, and Andrew. People told me that having a grandchild would be terrific, but I had no idea how terrific it would be. Speaking totally objectively, Nathaniel is the most terrific grandchild ever born, anywhere, anytime, ever.

Nathaniel extends my horizon. He will probably see the twenty-second century. Laptop computers will feel the same to him as typewriters do to me—quaint and useless. Maybe he'll see a colony on Mars. Maybe, a peaceful Middle East.

What will Nathaniel's America be like? Fact is, we don't know yet.

That's because Nathaniel is born at an American cusp—a time of choice. And, like it or not, the choices we're making about health care right now are going to hand Nathaniel the cards he'll be dealing with when most of us in this room won't be around anymore.

Like it or not, health care is now a big chapter in the story of global macroeconomics. This isn't just about whether we can afford universal coverage; it's about the whole country's fate. In 2011, the US national debt is going to surpass our entire gross domestic product—over $15 trillion. We're handing those cards to my grandson. If confidence falls in the economic health of America, then the vast numbers of American dollars in foreign hands fall in value. Other nations will seek other reserve currencies. Our standard of living will fall, and so will our capacity to invest—publicly or privately. And a key culprit, the biggest engine of decline, is the rising cost of health care, like it or not.

Sometimes people say, "Don't talk about costs and financial performance. That will demoralize health care workers; doctors won't like it. Stick to clinical quality." That won't cut it. Yes, we should celebrate our successes in technical care improvement, and never, never let up on them. But, the Forum is twenty-one years old—the quality movement is grown up. Health care and *macro*economics are now bonded for the long haul and we have to deal with that. If we, in improvement, ignore that linkage, we'll be dinosaurs. We'll be irrelevant to a massive, looming social need. The good news is that we can help—for sure, big time. To do that, we only have to think bigger. We have to think, as Rosabeth Moss Kanter says it, "Not just out of the box, but out of the building."

Let's start with a diagnosis. What's going on?

Last summer, President Obama seemed to shift his wording from "health care reform" to "health *insurance* reform." He was being accurate. That's what Congress is aiming for—better coverage, and changes in the rules and funding for coverage. The price is close to a trillion dollars over the next ten years, and there's a big debate about how to get that done. The debate is mainly about how to balance two options: find more money, or do less for people. Spend more, or help less.

But, neither of those plans—neither "spend more" nor "help less"—is going to work; not for long, and definitely not for Nathaniel. I cannot imagine that a civilized, developed country will actually deny highly effective and humane care to its people—that we'll say to Americans, "Too bad. Medical science has what you need, but you can't get it." But, I can't imagine, either, an America that just keeps spending more and more and more of its income on health care—16 percent, 20 percent, 25 percent. That's theft—theft by health care from schools and roads and museums and the social safety net. That's theft from the future. That's ripping off Nathaniel. We can't spend more on care, and we can't do less for people. But, that's a pickle. That's a mega-pickle.

How did we get into this fix? Well, politics did it. Politics forced us to cobble together a coalition of self-interest that's enough to pass a law that will get more people covered. Getting everyone covered is right; it's moral. We need that law, and we ought to pass it. Period. But, that doesn't change care. It doesn't make health care any better, any more valuable, or any more affordable. Remember? Every system is perfectly designed to achieve exactly the results it gets. You can't get new, better results at new, lower costs without a new system of care.

Congress hasn't led us to a new care system, and I don't think it will. Congress won't give America even a vague prescription, much less a detailed set of rules, for *that*. How could they? How could Congress possibly know enough to specify, for every community, the exact design for that: care that is safe, effective, patient-centered, timely, efficient, and equitable?

We're stuck. We're after a political compromise that gives more people care. That's good. But that won't give us the care we need or the care we can afford. That's bad. Where we're stuck isn't new. And it's not about health care. The problem is as old as human endeavor.

We're stuck in the "Tragedy of the Commons"—Garrett Hardin's term from his famous 1968 article in *Science*. Hardin imagined a pasture held in common by a community—anyone can graze his sheep there. There is an optimum number of grazing sheep for that Commons—fewer won't take full advantage of the grass, but too many will overgraze—they'll destroy the Commons. So, Hardin asks, "What does a rational person do?" Here's what a rational person does: add a sheep—over and over again, everybody adds sheep. Why? Because every individual gets his whole sheep, but the harm he does to the Commons is spread over the whole community. Anyone who individually limits his herd is a chump; he's a sucker; he's just giving up what everyone else is getting. "Therein is the tragedy," Hardin wrote. "Each man is locked into a system that compels him to increase his herd without limit—in a world that is limited. Ruin is the destination toward which all men rush. . . ."

Obviously, the Tragedy of the Commons isn't just about sheep. It's a threat whenever the smart strategy for each reasonable person separately is *not* the best strategy for all reasonable people together—when what's good for me isn't good for us.

It's about air and water and forests and traffic on the roads and where to dump nuclear waste. And now, it's about health care reform—in spades.

Like the villagers, rational health care stakeholders are eroding the common good simply by doing what makes sense to each of them—separately. In the short term, we each win. But, in the long term, we all lose. We lose the Triple Aim: better care for individuals, better health for populations, and lower per capita cost, all at once.

Name any stakeholder—hospital, physician, nurse, insurer, pharmaceutical manufacturer, supplier, even patients' groups—every single one of them says, "Oh, we need change! We need change!" But, when it comes to specifics, every single one of them demands to be kept whole or made better off. "Don't stop my sheep; stop his." So everybody draws on the Commons, the herds grow, and the Commons fails. If you don't increase your herd, you're a chump. And, who wants to be a chump?

Does it matter? Yes, it matters. It matters to Nathaniel, and Nathaniel matters to me. For Nathaniel, a bankrupt Medicare trust fund, a contracting economy, global warming, global poverty, failed states, and failing infrastructures aren't theoretical threats—they are the facts—

we're handing him those facts. We're saying, "Hey, Nathaniel, deal with it!" The Commons is Nathaniel's Commons; we're just trustees. We will be gone; he will be here.

This is a world with limits. It can be used up. And health care is exerting its claim on those limits beyond its right—beyond its needs. Health care is not entitled to everything it has, and *surely* not entitled to everything it can get.

Now, let me tell you something magical. Health care does not *need* everything it can get—not by a long shot, not if what it's trying to do is give *us* what *we* need—comfort, answers, vigor, years—health. We *can* have what we want. I know that sounds crazy after just speaking to you about limits, but I am sure it's true. But, we have to ask first, "What *do* we want?"

So, let's play a little game. I learned it from my colleague, Jay Ogilvie, who learned it from a psychologist named Jean Houston.

I want you to answer a question: When it comes to your health and your health care, what do you want?

Now, I have another question: When it comes to your health and your health care, what do you *really* want?

And, now, I have just one more question: When it comes to your health and your health care, what do you *really, really* want?

Can I tell you what I really, really want? To understand, you'll need some background.

First, cross-country skiing. I learned to skate ski when I lived in Anchorage, Alaska, for a year—1996 to 1997. Skate skiing is hard to learn. It is totally flailing, frustrating, falling. But, if you practice, after a long time it begins to click—it's a pendulum motion, very fluid; you attend to details of balance and shifting weight. In a hundred strokes, maybe three go right, and, for those three strokes, you fly—it's the closest I have ever felt to flying—through crisp winter air on five-meter-wide, rolling, forest trails. Then it is ten strokes in a hundred; then twenty-five. I'll tell you when I get to thirty.

Second, a birch grove in Waterville Valley, New Hampshire, where my family has a cabin; we go there every weekend we can. There are fifty kilometers of groomed skate skiing trails in Waterville Valley. Osceola Trail leads onto Moose Run, and four kilometers from Depot Camp, where you park your car, just across a stream and up a small hill, Moose Run trail winds gently for just a hundred meters or so through a small stand of young birch trees—white birch, gray birch, and black birch, all together. I don't know any lovelier spot in the world. If you are lucky, and no other skiers happen by for a few minutes, you can stop there, and stand still, and lean on your ski poles in the silence, and watch a busy red squirrel, and feel totally at peace.

In 2003, six Forums ago, I gave a plenary speech about a problem I have—in my right knee. The problem is osteoarthritis, from botched surgery when I was a medical student, aggravated by years of jogging. In December 2004, in bad pain, I was just about to have a total knee replacement. But, at the last minute, a week before surgery, an orthopedist—a third opinion—suggested trying a steroid injection in my knee. My surgeon agreed to try, and, here I am, five years—and just one more steroid shot—later, limping a little, but almost pain free, and with my own knee still there. It's not perfect. I can't jog even a single step; I have to wear special orthotics; when I hike, I have to use poles to take some weight. But, and here is the important point, I *can* skate ski—all I want. With a metal knee, I probably couldn't; it can't take the torque. And, guess what—snow just fell in Waterville Valley, and, if it sticks, next weekend I'll be up there, quiet, on Moose Run, leaning on my ski poles, watching a little red squirrel watching me.

What health care do I want? Of course, what I want is safe, effective, evidence-based health care for my knee. But, what I *really* want is to skate ski on that knee. But, what I *really, really* want is five minutes on a sun-filled, blue-skied, 20-degree, February afternoon in total silence, leaning on my ski poles in that little stand of birches watching one busy red squirrel.

Now, I'm not saying that I won't need a metal knee someday; I probably will. But, just not yet. Not yet. Health care wanted to give me a metal knee, and was all too ready to move; I wanted to visit a squirrel. My care was dignified and professional, but it missed the point. And I can't help wondering what my health care would be like if it *understood* the point: that it's not what health care *does* that matters, but rather how well it helps us with our deepest, realest needs—how it touches our souls.

I am going to take a guess. I doubt that any single person here—when you got down to what you *really, really* want—named any health care at all. Nobody *really, really* wants a doctor visit, or a blood test, or a CT scan, or a night in a hospital. I know what you really, really want. You want Thanksgiving dinner with your family, or quiet time with your partner, or a soft chair and a great book, or a dive into the cool water. You want two more fly casts before the sun sets, to see that van Gogh, or to hear that chorale one more time, see that view from the summit. Me, I really, really want to teach Nathaniel to skate ski, and to introduce him to a squirrel.

Health care has no intrinsic value at all. None. None. Health does. Joy does. Peace does.

What, in heaven's name, does that have to do with health care reform, and macroeconomics, and the Medicare trust fund, and Nathaniel's future?

Everything. A health care system that gave us each what we *really, really* want would be—it *can* be—a system sustainable for our futures and for our children's futures. It is different from the one we have. The best health care is the very, very least health care that we need to gain the long, full, and joyous lives that we really, really want. The best hospital bed is empty, not full. The best CT scan is the one we don't need to take. The best doctor's visit is the one we don't need to have.

We are trying to change. We are groping toward change with technical terms and initiatives, like value-based purchasing, evidence-based care, Lean production, or, even Triple Aim. But, a better term might be this: "getting what we really, really want." To find it, we have to escape from the Tragedy of the Commons. We have to escape from the instinct simply to keep and grow what we have, simply to do what we do, and instead to embrace curiosity about the meaning, the purpose, the *why*.

When we don't ask, we hurt the Commons. I'm sure you read Atul Gawande's barrier-shattering article in the *New Yorker* magazine this year, the one about McAllen, Texas. Atul used the *Dartmouth Atlas* to find McAllen. The Dartmouth Atlas Project uses Medicare data and sectors the United States into 306 regions—hospital referral regions, or HRRs—to study patterns of expenditure and quality across those regions. Only the Miami, Florida, HRR is more costly per capita than McAllen is. Incredibly, McAllen's per capita Medicare cost—$15,000—is $3,000 per year higher than its per capita income. Yet, McAllen isn't any better at all in quality, outcomes, or service to the people of that HRR than lots of HRRs that cost much less.

This summer, Atul, Elliott Fisher, Maureen Bisognano, Tom Nolan, Mark McClellan, and I got together to study the other end of the curve— the lowest cost HRRs. We found 74 of the 306 that were in the lowest quartile of cost and had above-average quality. They have average costs of about $8,000 per year, compared with McAllen's $15,000. In fact, they're 16 percent below the US *average*.

We called our project, "How Do They Do That?" We wanted to know. We picked ten of these high-performing communities and invited them to send teams to come to D.C. for a meeting this past July.

These ten are a pretty good slice of America. In fact, that's how we chose them: Everett, Washington; Temple, Texas; Asheville, North

Carolina; Richmond, Virginia; Sayre, Pennsylvania; Portland, Maine; Sacramento, California; La Crosse, Wisconsin; Tallahassee, Florida; and Cedar Rapids, Iowa. They're sort of "normal," except for how they use health care resources. In that, they're abnormal. Overall, at least for Medicare, they use hospital days 15 percent less than average, specialist visits 30 percent less, and images 25 percent less. Their quality scores and patient satisfaction are mostly well above average. If the whole United States looked like these places, we wouldn't have a health care crisis. We could have universal coverage, better outcomes, higher satisfaction, and lots of money left over to spend on public health, education, roads, museums, or whatever else we wanted.

How *do* they do that? We're not sure yet, but we think we see patterns. And the most impressive pattern of all—the one I think that's going to come out at the top—is cooperation, founded on respect for the community as a whole—a sense of the Commons.

I could talk about any of them, but I am going to pick on Cedar Rapids, Iowa. Cedar Rapids doesn't look very much like Zorko in Ghana, and Jim Levett, a cardiac surgeon and CMO of the multispecialty group in town, looks nothing at all like Hajia Mary Issaka. Neither, for that matter, do Tim Charles or Ted Townsend, the CEOs of the two competing hospitals in town—Mercy and St. Luke's. But, I have a sneaking suspicion that Mary, Jim, Tim, and Ted might hit it off if they met. They'd discover how much stock they put in "respect." For Mary, it's respect for each woman who comes for help. For these Cedar Rapids leaders, it's respect for the community they share—for Cedar Rapids's Commons.

Does Cedar Rapids have a Commons? That's a tough question. Let me answer it two ways.

First, I'd claim, Cedar Rapids has a health care Commons. Every health care provider—anyone who can spend a health care dollar—puts sheep on that Commons and draws it down. When they do that, somebody, somewhere, loses the chance to spend that dollar somewhere else on health care—if the pool is limited. It is limited. Medicare doesn't want to spend more, and, if you read those House and Senate bills, it looks like it's about to spend quite a bit less. And, the big employers in Cedar Rapids don't want private health insurance rates to go up; that would make it harder for them to find workers and to stay competitive. So, Jim and Tim and Ted and their colleagues have sort of a common budget, even if they never really add it up or try to manage it together: it's the total amount of money Cedar Rapids can get to fund care—to seek health. If a Cedar Rapids doctor orders a ton of CT scans, that's sheep on the Commons; if one of the hospitals adds beds or jacks up the admission rate, those are sheep on the Commons. It means that something else good for health won't get done.

But, there is a second way to think of the Commons there—a bigger Commons in which health care, itself, is only one sheep. That bigger Commons is Cedar Rapids's overall vitality as a community—its capacity to invest in good things *other than health care* for the 130,000 people who live there. That's reflected, for example, in wages. Between 1999 and 2009 in the United States, average family health insurance premiums went up 131 percent, while salaries and benefits rose only 37 percent. What does that mean if you work in Cedar Rapids and your salary is, say, $80,000 a year? You and your employer are now paying $13,000 of that—16 percent—for insurance, and more out of pocket. That's your money. If Cedar Rapids's health care looked like, say, Denmark's health care, that cost would be 8 percent of your pay, or $6,500. What could you do with an extra $6,500 a year? Of course, if Cedar Rapids looked like McAllen, Texas, you'd be a lot worse off.

If you're a Cedar Rapids city manager, part of that bigger Commons is the pool available for public investments—parks, public safety, Fourth of July fireworks, and pupil-to-teacher ratios. Reduce health care costs—more teachers. Raise health care costs—forget that new park. If you're an employer there, the Commons covers what you can pay your workers and how attractive your city is to new businesses. Raise health care costs—a worse deal for the workforce of the future. Reduce health care costs—Cedar Rapids's economy grows.

Yes, Cedar Rapids has a Commons, where health care grazes its sheep. "It's our money," Tom Nolan says.

Now, by some measures, Cedar Rapids looks pretty good when it comes to managing its Commons. Health care there actually costs about 27 percent less than in the average US community, according to the *Dartmouth Atlas*. For Medicare beneficiaries, they spend about $6,054 per person—compared with a US average of $8,304—and the quality of care is just about as high as any we can find in our country. Somebody, somewhere in Cedar Rapids seems to be counting the sheep.

Who? What's going on? Not sure. When you talk with Ted and Tim and Jim, they seem to describe cooperation. The doctors are a free-standing group, but they constantly work with the hospitals on quality and improvement. They study their own utilization patterns; they create their own protocols and stick by them. The hospitals compete, but they also cooperate. They're *this close* to agreeing to have only one cancer center in town, because the town needs only one. They have only one cardiac surgery program—that way they get better results and lower costs. There's even some talk of creating a unified structure—Ted Townsend calls it a "public utility" structure—to manage the care right across the continuum, and substitute planning for competition. And, maybe it's not an accident that, when you talk to these people, they sound proud of their town. They tell you how good life is in Cedar Rapids. They say people care. When the flood struck, everybody helped.

But, don't be naïve. They could lose their way. It's scary to see how easy it would be for Cedar Rapids today to become McAllen tomorrow —in a heartbeat, actually. The physician group is building its own 180,000-square-foot, $40 million medical building—right between the two hospitals. Will they do a little ambulatory surgery there? And then more? And then a whole lot more? The hospitals have different owner- ship structures. Will their boards go along with shared services? Or, will they say, "Wait a minute, my father helped build this place! We need one of our own." When a new group comes into town and revs up its own CT scanner, will the people of Cedar Rapids say, "Finally. We can get a scan anytime we want—that's quality," and go there, forcing the hospital and the doctors to do more scans themselves to keep up? Or, will the medical leaders speak up, earn trust, and explain to the people of Cedar Rapids that more is not always better in health care. Will they tell them that one CT scan of the abdomen is the same radiation expo- sure as four hundred chest X-rays, and that maybe less, not more, is better?

Cooperation—respect—sensible governance of the Commons—is alive in Cedar Rapids. And I could just as well have described dozens of other American communities—Everett, La Crosse, Tallahassee, and Port- land would have suited me fine. But, let me tell you, success in Cedar Rapids, and in Everett, La Crosse, Tallahassee, and Portland—respect for the Commons—hangs by a thread. It hangs by a thread. That's the thread that somehow in these places keeps the sense of the Commons, itself, alive. It's the thread that lets competitors cross no-man's-land and meet and talk, and keep meeting and keep talking. It's the thread that somehow lets Jim Levett continue to believe, and continue to say, that we're all in this together, and that the hospitals and the doctors are not natural enemies, but common villagers. It's the thread that connects leaders more firmly to their legacy than to their quarterly report, and that welcomes constraints—that *creates* constraints—so that "more sheep, more sheep, more sheep" isn't even available as an answer. I will go so far as to say that it is the thread of affection—love, maybe—for the idea that there *is* a Cedar Rapids, and that it is a common home, with a common will, and much good to do. And that something very important there is also very fragile and limited, and could be lost.

I don't blame Washington for leaving health care redesign to us. I don't think it's Washington's job. I think it's ours. The care we need—the system we want—will not come from what they do; it will come from what we do. Cedar Rapids isn't reading someone else's rule book; they're writing their own.

There is actually theory for this: governing the Commons. This year, Elinor Ostrom became the first woman ever to win the Nobel Prize for economics. *Governing the Commons* is the title of her key 1990 book. Professor Ostrom is a student of problems of collective action. She is out to solve the Tragedy of the Commons.

That's why she won the Nobel Prize. She has spent decades finding and studying real communities—communities that manage what she calls "common pool resources" effectively and escape from the tragedy, and those that don't. She has studied fisheries, forests, irrigation canals, bridges, parking lots, lakes, shared mainframe computers, and, yes, real grazing lands.

Take the fishermen of Alanya, Turkey. Fish are a common pool resource—they can be depleted, the resource as a whole cannot be easily owned, and its product can be appropriated—the fish I catch you can't catch. The hundred or so fishermen of Alanya work in two- or three-person boats. Each year, the community prepares a list of eligible boats. They name and list the good fishing spots. In September, the eligible boats draw lots to assign a fishing spot to each. And then, each day from September to January, each boat moves east to the next spot. From January to May, each boat moves west each day, equalizing the effects of the direction of fish migration. The fishermen monitor the system themselves; obviously they'll know right away if one of them hasn't moved, or is cheating. Nobody told the people of Alanya to do that; they made up their own rules. Professor Ostrom would say that they created their own "institution" (that's her word)—their own rule book—to protect the Commons.

Professor Ostrom refuses to accept that the Tragedy of the Commons is fated. She says, "I would rather address the question of how to enhance the capabilities of those involved to change the constraining rules of the game to lead to outcomes other than remorseless tragedies." I repeat: "to change the constraining rules of the game to lead to outcomes other than remorseless tragedies."

Professor Ostrom has studied many groups like the fishermen of Alanya. And she has found a few common design principles in groups that successfully avoid the "remorseless tragedy":

- They know their boundaries. They know who is using the common resource, and they know the limits of what they have.

- They make rules that fit the local context. Their rules for use of the Commons are their own, not handed down from remote authorities.

- They decide together. The people affected by the rules can have voice in changing them.

- They measure and monitor. They actively audit their own behaviors and resource conditions.

- They can be tough. They create and use sanctions. They create consequences, swift and local, for people who violate the rules.

- They have ways to confront and resolve conflicts, when they occur—as they always do—at low cost.

- And, very importantly, they have sufficient latitude to act. External governmental authorities don't challenge their right to devise their own institutions to govern the Commons locally.

I don't know if the people of Cedar Rapids, Everett, Washington, Portland, or La Crosse know Elinor Ostrom's work; but she'd recognize theirs. These are communities managing a common pool resource—health care. They are not waiting for instruction, not waiting for external authority to rescue them from the trap. They are rescuing themselves.

It isn't easy. Positive collective action, even in small communities, and especially in health care, is fragile. It could all just fall apart. But, it can work. I know it *can* work because, sometimes, some places, it *does* work.

Cedar Rapids, La Crosse, Everett, Tallahassee, Grand Junction, Portland—these are not on the moon or in a galaxy far, far away. They are among us and there is no good reason on Earth that we can't follow their lead.

Here is my challenge. I challenge us to end the Tragedy of the Commons in health care. I challenge us to prove Garrett Hardin wrong. I challenge us to be as wise as the fishermen of Alanya. I challenge Cedar Rapids, not just to succeed, but to *continue* to succeed. And, I hope for McAllen, Texas; I challenge McAllen to learn and change.

But, I'm very mindful of who you all are. You are doctors and nurses tending patients, operating room managers trying to keep 6 West going or clear the waiting lines. You're QI directors coaxing the operating room into using a checklist, or executives getting ready to tell the board some bad news. And, I think, you're wondering, "What can I do from my limited perch to govern the Commons better? I'm already over my head."

I am really not sure. But, I have a strong feeling that it can—it has to—start with you. Command-and-control solutions seem weaker every day, and Elinor Ostrom's brilliant explorations suggest that, in many contexts, higher authorities simply can't do the job. Maybe someone smart enough and courageous enough in Washington can write a few rules that change the odds—in fact, we need some tough rules from Washington that make it hard—impossible, maybe—to simply go on with business as usual. But, the odds of real reform, "re-form," remain zero—the Commons is doomed—unless the action is closer to home— closer to you. So, drawing on Elinor Ostrom's work, here are some ideas to start chewing on.

1. *Understand your health care Commons.* Understand its limits and boundaries. Understand who can and does draw upon the common pool of resources, and who it serves.

2. *Adopt an aim.* Here's one: Over the next three years, reduce the total resource consumption of your health care system, no matter where you start, by 10 percent. Do this without a single instance of harm, rationing of effective care, or exclusion of needed services for the population you serve. Do it by focusing not on the habits of health care as it is now, but by focusing on what really, really matters. Amory Lovins calls it "end use efficiency." I call it "a squirrel." I'll mention, too, that Tom Nolan and I have been working hard on a framework for better care at lower cost— that 10 percent goal—a driver diagram for better care at lower cost.

3. *Develop, fast, because there isn't much time left, your own institutional structures*—the ones you will need for local rule-making to better manage your common pool resource. Do *not* wait for external rules to be made, or to change; do it yourself. One such structure might be, for example, a community-wide board— the collection together of all the health care boards with shared stewardship of the whole.

4. *Develop, fast, because there isn't much time left, monitors, so that you can track the use of the common resource*, and find out who is sticking to the rules you write, and who is breaking them.

5. *When people do break the rules—opportunists, free riders—create undesirable consequences for them*, if you can, and ways to isolate them, if you cannot. Collective action is very fragile. You will need militia.

6. *Identify and address conflicts early, often, and with confidence.*
Conflicts will be frequent and legitimate, and they will demand
wisdom. The social capital—the commitment to protect the
Commons—has got to trump these conflicts.

7. *Expect and offer civility.* This is the foundational transactional rule
for effective, collaborative management of what we hold in trust.
Remember Hajia Mary Issaka in Ghana. Respect is a precondition.

When I was a child, I waited to be helped. My mother woke me for
school. My lunch was packed. I had a bedtime. It was nice. It wasn't
freedom, but it was nice.

Now, it's on me. I pack lunch. It's hard work—judgments to make,
decisions, choices, folding clothes. I'm freer, but I have to earn my way.

You know what I think? I think we're twenty-one. I think it's grown-up
time. I think we get one life, and that waiting for solutions to the insanity
of health care that costs too much and achieves too little is getting a little
boring and old-hat. I think that prom night is over. I think it's time to
cook our own meals, and make our own beds, and set our own sails,
and pick our own destinations, and make our own, wise rules. And I
think the first of those rules has to be the rule of respect—respect for the
Commons; respect for the needs of the patient and of the community
that we share with the patient; respect for both limits and possibility;
and respect for ourselves—for our creativity and ingenuity and good
will—and *tough* good will.

Nathaniel needs this. Whether we can find the will and wisdom to
work our way, as communities, out of the trap of the Tragedy of the
Commons has everything to do with the world Nathaniel is going to live
in and grow old in. Cedar Rapids's Commons hangs by a thread. And,
on that very same thread hangs the future of my grandson.

My friends, we can spend our days ahead fighting for our piece of the
pie. We have plenty of role models for that. But, that's for summer camp
and the schoolyard; not for here. Not for this real and fragile world. Not
for the Commons. Not when there is only one pie, and it is all we have
and all we will ever have, and it is in our hands to preserve—not just
for us, but for our children and our grandchildren. We can wait for the
rules to be written by others and for the laws on tablets chiseled by others
to rescue us, but those rules will be less wise than the ones we can write,
and those tablets will be, not our salvation, but weights upon our spirit.
It is a very tough choice. Get everything we can? Or, respect everything
we have been given?

Chapter 12

YOU DECIDE

COMMENTARY

Beverley H. Johnson

IN HIS ELOQUENT speech at the Yale School of Medicine
graduation in 2010, Don Berwick challenged the graduates to
"unlock the door" of policy and rules to open health care
to participation by patients and families. He shared stories
from his personal and professional experience to inspire the
students to make this choice.

Family presence is a theme woven throughout the stories in
Dr. Berwick's speech. His daughter was one of the graduates,
and he spoke about the memory of his presence at her
birth—and the importance of that opportunity. He also
shared his expectation for care at the end of life, explaining
how he would want to spend time together with his wife,
reliving their shared memories.

Dr. Berwick also shared Jackie Gruzenski's story of being
separated from her husband during the last days of his life.
Mrs. Gruzenski described her husband, a psychiatrist, as a
very good doctor and a very good husband. He knew he had
a serious life-threatening illness, and he had planned the way
he wanted to be cared for at the end of his life. But the
physicians and nurses who cared for him used their "power
and privilege" to invoke policies that caused harm and
distress to both Dr. and Mrs. Gruzenski. The rules labeled
Mrs. Gruzenski a visitor; Dr. Gruzenski's repeated response
was, "She is not a visitor, she is my wife."

Dr. Berwick explained that he did not share this story to "sadden" the students, but to inspire them to make a choice, rather than be controlled by "deaf habit." This was a powerful message for the next generation of physicians to respect the preferences and preserve the dignity of patients and their families.

Dr. Berwick's stories have meaning for all in health care. Rachel Naomi Remen, the physician author of *Kitchen Table Wisdom: Stories That Heal*, has said that "facts bring us to knowledge; stories bring us to wisdom." We know, too, that a characteristic of high-performing health care organizations is the ability of the leaders to share stories. With stories, you can engage the hearts and minds of physicians and all health care professionals, to strive for excellence in all domains of practice.

With the sharing of Mrs. Gruzenski's story, Dr. Berwick issues a call for action to address a major flaw in today's health care system: labeling families as visitors in policy and practice, imposing inhumane restrictions on family access to their loved ones during a hospital stay, causing isolation for patients often at times of their greatest vulnerability, and placing patients at risk for harm. These policies and practices must change.

A message for experienced leaders and front-line staff in hospitals, as well as new physicians, is the importance of respecting how patients define their families and how they want them to be involved in care and decision making. Both practitioners and health care organizations should use a broad definition of family to guide their vision, policies, and practices. The Memorial Healthcare System in Hollywood, Florida, has developed this definition of family for their health system: "The term 'family' has many meanings and includes not only traditional bonds created by marriages and common ancestry, but also bonds created by close friendships, commitments, shared households, shared children-rearing responsibilities, and romantic attachments." The American Academy of Family Physicians defines family as "a group of individuals with a continuing legal, genetic and/or emotional relationship."

There is no evidence that considering family members "visitors" and establishing restrictive "visiting" hours is the right thing to do. In fact, the evidence is compelling that welcoming and supporting families as care partners according to patient preference has many benefits for patients and families, for staff and clinicians, and for the health care organization.

Dr. Berwick also speaks of the role of healers, aligning with the continuous healing relationships described in the landmark Institute of Medicine report, *Crossing the Quality Chasm*. The role of healers is grounded in partnership—ensuring respect and dignity, sharing information in useful and affirming ways, and encouraging participation of patients and families in care and decision making. These are the core concepts of patient- and family-centered care. An essential practice of patient- and family-centered care is welcoming and supporting family presence and participation in all health care settings.

Now is the time to change the concept of families as visitors and to move toward respecting and encouraging families in their essential caring roles and recognizing them as allies for quality and safety.

YOU DECIDE

YALE SCHOOL OF MEDICINE GRADUATION ADDRESS
NEW HAVEN, CONNECTICUT, MAY 24, 2010

DEAN ALPERN, FACULTY, families, friends, and honored graduates . . .

I don't have words enough to express my gratitude for the chance to speak with you on your special day. It would be a pleasure and honor at any graduation ceremony. But, I have to tell you, to be up here in this role in the presence of my own daughter on the day that she becomes a doctor is a joy I wouldn't dare have dreamed up. I hope that each of you will someday have the chance to feel as much gratitude and pride and love as I feel right now, joining you, and, especially, joining Jessica. Thank you very much. I am so proud of you, Jessica.

Now, I have to tell you the truth about Jessica. Jessica was supposed to be a boy. At least that's what the ultrasonographer said when we took a look at "him" in utero. "Never been wrong," said the ultrasound tech as she pointed out the anatomy—there was the "thing." My wife and I were delighted. We saw the thing, too. Clearly. We had two sons already, and they were fantastic. A third boy—terrific!

But, you know, to be honest, and with no offense intended to Ben and Dan, who are here today, too, we were sort of hoping for a change. I had only brothers, and Ann, my wife, I knew, wanted a chance to raise a daughter. To our friends we said, "Boy . . . Girl . . . We don't care; just as long as he is healthy." But. . . we were lying, just a little.

And then: the surprise. I was right *there*, in the c-section room—Ann delivered all four of our children by c-section—and, instead of Jonas, whom we were waiting for, out popped, not Jonas, but Jessica. "Oh, my goodness," the obstetrician exclaimed, "it's a girl!" Imagine the joy—Ann and I literally squealed. We screamed. "A daughter," Ann screamed, "a daughter . . . We have a daughter!"

The obstetrician said, "Hmmmm . . . That never happened before. That 'thing' on the ultrasound must have been the umbilical cord." Whatever. No question at all—that was one of the peak moments of my entire life. I will never, ever forget it. I had a daughter.

How do I know that moment of miracle—that surprise and celebration? Well, it's obvious. I told you. I was *there*—I was right *there* in the c-section room, holding my wife's hand. Greeting my new, unexpected daughter. *Watching* the miracle.

Maybe you know this; maybe you don't. But, if that had happened twenty years before Jessica was born, or even ten, I would have missed it. I wouldn't have been there. I *couldn't* have been there, because fathers weren't allowed in c-section rooms. We weren't supposed to be there. That was the rule. Then, somebody changed the rule; somebody courageous, I suspect. And, so, I got to see a miracle.

Let me read to you an email I received on Thursday, December 19, 2009. It came from Mrs. Jocelyn Anne Gruzenski—she goes by "Jackie." I did not know Jackie Gruzenski at the time; she wrote to me out of the blue. But I have since connected with her. And, she gave me permission to read her email to me to you. Here's what she wrote:

> Dr. Berwick,
>   . . . My husband was Dr. William Paul Gruzenski, a psychiatrist for 39 years. He was admitted to [a hospital she names in Pennsylvania] after developing a cerebral bleed with a hypertensive crisis. My issue is that I was denied access to my husband except for very strict visiting, 4 times a day for 30 minutes, and that my husband was hospitalized behind a locked door. My husband and I were rarely separated except for work. . . . He wanted me present in the ICU, and he challenged the ICU nurse and MD saying, "She is not a visitor, she is my wife." But, it made no difference. My husband was in the ICU for eight days out of his last 16 days alive, and there were a lot of missed opportunities for us.

Mrs. Gruzenski continued:

> I am advocating to the hospital administration that visiting hours have to be open, especially for spouses. . . . I do not feel that his care was individualized to meet his needs; he wanted me there more than I was allowed. I feel it was a very cruel thing that was done to us. . . .

Listen, again, to the words of Dr. Gruzenski: "She is not a visitor, she is my wife." Hear, again, Mrs. Gruzenski: "I feel it was a very cruel thing that was done to us."

Cruel is a powerful word for Mrs. Gruzenski to use, isn't it? Her email and the emails that followed that first one are without exception dignified, respectful, tempered. Why does she say "cruel"?

We will have to imagine ourselves there. "My husband and I loved each other very deeply," she writes to me, "and we wanted to share our last days and moments together. We both knew the gravity of his illness, and my husband wanted quality of life, not quantity."

What might a husband and wife of nineteen years, aware of the short time left together, wish to talk about—wish to do—in the last days? I don't know for Dr. and Mrs. Gruzenski. But, I do know for me. I would talk about our children. I would talk about the best trip we ever took together, and even argue, smiling, about whose idea it was. I would remember the black bear we met in a clearing in the Wrangell-St. Elias Range; the cabin at Assiniboine; the Jøtenheim mountains of Norway. I would remember being lost in Kyoto and lost in Prague and lost on Mount Washington, and always found again. Mushroom soup at Café Budapest. And seeing Jessica born, and Ben, and Dan, and Becca. We would have so much to talk about. So much. The nurses would pad in and out of the hospital room, checking IVs and measuring pulses and planning their dinners and their weekends. And none of what the nurses and doctors did would matter to us at all; we wouldn't even notice them. We would know exactly who the visitors were—they, the doctors and the nurses. They, they would be the visitors in this tiny corner of our whole lives together—they, not us. In the John Denver song it goes this way, "And all the time that you're with me, we will be at home."

Someone stole all of that from Dr. and Mrs. Gruzenski. A nameless someone. I suspect an unknowing someone. Someone who did not understand who was at home and who was the guest—who was the intruder. Someone who forgot about the black bear and the best mushroom soup we ever had—the jewels of shared experience that glimmer with meaning in our lives. Someone who put the IV first, and the soul second.

Of course, it isn't really "someone" at all. We don't even know who, or what it is. Its voice sounds rational. Its words are these: "It is our policy," "It's against the rule," "It would be a problem," and even, incredibly, "It is in your own best interest." What is irrational is not those phrases; they seem to make sense. What is irrational is what follows those phrases, in ellipsis, unsaid: "It is our policy . . . that you cannot hold your husband's hand." "It is against the rules . . . to let you see this or to let you know this." "It would be a problem . . . if we treated you on your own terms not ours." "It is in your own best interest . . . to miss your daughter's moment of birth." This is the voice of power; and power does not always think the whole thing through. Power, even when it has no name and no locus, power can be, to borrow Mrs. Gruzenski's word, "cruel."

I want you to celebrate this day. I want you to experience all of the pride, all of the joy that it brings you to have reached this milestone. I am not telling you Dr. and Mrs. Gruzenski's story to sadden you. I am telling it to inspire you. I want you to remember it, if you can possibly remember anything I am saying to you at this chock-full moment of your lives, because that story gives you a choice.

You see, today you take a big step into power. With your white coat and your Latin, with your anatomy lessons and your stethoscope, you enter today a life of new and vast privilege. You may not notice your power at first. You will not always feel powerful or privileged—not when you are filling out endless billing forms and swallowing requirements and struggling through hard days of too many tasks. But this will be true: In return for your years of learning and your dedication to a life of service and your willingness to take an oath to that duty, society will give you access and rights that it gives to no one else. Society will allow you to hear secrets from frightened human beings that they are too scared to tell anyone else. Society will permit you to use drugs and instruments that can do great harm as well as great good, and that in the hands of others would be weapons. Society will give you special titles and spaces of privilege, as if you were priests. Society will let you build walls and write rules.

And in that role, with that power, you will meet Dr. and Mrs. Gruzenski over, and over, and over again. You will meet them every day—every hour. They will be in disguise. They will be disguised as a new mother afraid to touch her premie on the ventilator in the incubator. Disguised as the construction worker too embarrassed to admit that he didn't hear a word you just said after, "It might be cancer." Disguised as the busy lawyer who cannot afford for you to keep her waiting, but too polite to say so. Disguised as the alcoholic bottoming out who was the handsome champion of his soccer team and dreamed of being an architect someday. Disguised as the child over whom you tower. Disguised as the ninety-year-old grandmother, over whom you tower. Disguised as the professor in the MRI machine who has been told to lie still, but who desperately needs to urinate and is ashamed. Disguised as the man who would prefer to know; and the man who would prefer *not* to know. Disguised as the woman who would prefer to sit; and as the woman who would prefer to stand. And as the man who wants you to call him, "Bill," and as the man who prefers to be called, "Dr. Gruzenski."

Mrs. Gruzenski wrote, "My husband was a very caring physician and administrator for many years, but during his hospitalization, he was not even afforded the respect of being called, 'Doctor.' " Dr. Gruzenski wanted to be called "Dr. Gruzenski." But, they did not do so.

You can. That choice is not in the hands of nameless power, not fated to control by deaf habit. Not "our policy," "the rule." Just you. Your choice. Your rule. Your power.

What is at stake here may seem a small thing in the face of the enormous health care world you have joined. It is as a nickel to the $2.6 trillion industry. But that small thing is what matters. I will tell you: it is *all* that matters. All that matters is the person. The person. The individual. The patient. The poet. The lover. The adventurer. The frightened soul. The wondering mind. The learned mind. The Husband. The Wife. The Son. The Daughter. In the moment.

In the moment, it is all about choice. You have a magical opportunity. You have the opportunity to decide. Yes, you can read the rule book; and someday you can even write the rule book. Decide. Yes, you can hide behind the protocols and the policies. Decide. Yes, you can say "we," when you mean, "I." Yes, you can lock the door. "Sorry, Mrs. Gruzenski, your thirty minutes are up." You can say that.

But, you can also *unlock* the door. You can ask, "Shall I call you 'Dr. Gruzenski'?" "Would you like to be alone?" "Is this a convenient time?" "Is there something else I can do for you?" You can say, "You're the boss." You can say, "Tell me about the best trip you ever took. Tell me about the time you saw your daughter born."

In my first week of medical school, I was assigned a tutor: Dr. Edward Frank. He was a vascular surgeon, and he was to supervise me in my physical diagnosis course. I read what Harvard Medical School called, "The Red Book." It was all about the history and physical exam. Hundreds of questions to ask—history, physical, chief complaint, review of systems, and on and on. I stayed up very late, studying all those questions; memorizing the ritual. I knew all the right questions, I thought. I met Dr. Frank the next afternoon, and he took me to see Mrs. Goldberg, who was in the hospital to have her gall bladder taken out. Dr. Frank brought me into Mrs. Goldberg's room, into her presence, introduced me, and invited me to begin. My very first history and physical.

"Tell me, Mrs. Goldberg," I said, "when did your pain begin?" Dr. Frank, the surgeon, interrupted me. He gently put his hand on my shoulder, and he gave me a gift I will never, ever forget. And I will pass his gift to you. His gift was a question that the Red Book left out.

"Oh, Don," he said. "Before you ask that, let me tell you something very special. Did you know that Mrs. Goldberg has a brand new grandson?"

Decide. You can read the rules. Or, you can say, "Pardon me." "Pardon this unwelcome interruption in your lives. Thank you for inviting me to help. Thank you for letting me visit. I am your guest, and I know it. Now, please, Mrs. Gruzenski, Dr. Gruzenski, what may I do for you?"

Congratulations on your achievement today. Feel proud. You ought to. When you put on your white coat, my dear friends, you become a doctor.

But, now I will tell you a secret—a mystery. Those who suffer need you to be something more than a doctor; they need you to be a healer. And, to become a healer, you must do something even more difficult than putting your white coat on. You must take your white coat off. You must recover, embrace, and treasure the memory of your shared, frail humanity—of the dignity in each and every soul. When you take off that white coat in the sacred presence of those for whom you will care—in the sacred presence of people just like you—when you take off that white coat, and, tower not over them, but join those you serve, you become a healer in a world of fear and fragmentation, an "aching" world, as your chaplain put it this morning, that has never needed healing more.

Congratulations.

Chapter 13

THE MORAL TEST

COMMENTARY

Tom Daschle

IT WAS IN October 1972, in a town called Webster, South
Dakota, that I first heard Senator Hubert Humphrey, a
South Dakotan by birth, define the moral test of government.
The test, he said, is "how it treats those who are in the dawn
of life, the children; those who are in the twilight of life, the
aged; and those in the shadows of life, the sick, the needy and
the handicapped."

It so moved me that I remember writing it down on a piece
of scrap paper that I had in my pocket. I have since repeated
it in hundreds of speeches, in scores of different contexts and
venues.

In more than forty years of public life, I have never come
across a more succinct or more accurate definition of the
moral test, not only of government, but, as Don Berwick
notes in the extraordinary speech you are about to read, the
nation. History will define Americans in large measure by
how successfully we meet it.

How fitting that this quotation is inscribed in the Hubert
Humphrey Building, the very heart of the Department of
Health and Human Services. And how appropriate it is that
Dr. Berwick considers it the inspiration for his thoughtful and
compelling speech on the transformative challenges we now
face in health care and the manner in which we should
address them.

My only regret is that Senator Humphrey's definition of our moral test is not inscribed in the US Capitol as well so that members of Congress, too, could be equally as motivated to use these words for their speeches in the chambers of both the Senate and House of Representatives.

How good it would be if every US senator and representative were admonished to remember them every time they walk through the historic Capitol doors and onto the floors of the two chambers where they cast their votes.

Yet perhaps I can say from personal experience, what members of Congress do, or don't do, must only be viewed as one of many factors in the ultimate determination of our success in meeting the moral test. There have been moments through history when Congress has risen magnificently to the occasion, giving our country the leadership it desperately needed. And there have been times when it has failed miserably.

However, in both sets of circumstances, it is the collective spirit and will of the American people, not just the actions of a president or Congress, that define an era and create the momentum for positive change and enlightened action.

And therein lies the message and the challenge to us all that Dr. Berwick so eloquently articulated in his speech at the IHI National Forum in December 2011. If we are to pass the moral test of this generation, in large measure, one critical set of criteria will be how accessible, how safe, and how cost-efficient health care will be for all Americans. And it is up to each of us involved in health care, in our own way, and with our own abilities and circumstances, to ensure that our country rises to this historic occasion.

With recognition and gratitude from millions of Americans for President Barack Obama's leadership, Congress enacted the Patient Protection and Affordable Care Act (PPACA) to create the framework for a new and necessary health care infrastructure. But the framework is only that. It creates the means by which, through effective leadership and action at all levels, we can build a more just, a more humane, and a more enduring society with high-performance, high-quality health care that incorporates better access, better quality, and lower cost.

There may be no better messenger for this collective call to action than Don Berwick. To the regret and deep disappointment of many of those Americans who lauded the president's leadership, Congress failed to confirm Dr. Berwick as Centers for Medicare & Medicaid Services (CMS) administrator. Yet, for seventeen months, he became one of the strongest, most compelling leaders for change as he motivated audiences, CMS employees, Congress, and the entire health sector at large. Then, having reached the expiration of his term in office, he has determinedly continued to practice what he preached, maintaining an active engagement and leadership role in the call for change in both health policy and practice.

There has never been a more dynamic, transformative moment for health care in America than the one we are experiencing now. Our success in making the most of it will be determined in large measure by our resiliency and our innovation. But it can also only be achieved through our willingness to collaborate by helping those who help others, and by the level of our active engagement in improving all aspects of our new health care universe. In effect, by how well we do it all.

In short, our success will depend upon our collective leadership and, most important, our ability to remember patients, especially those patients in the dawn, twilight, and shadows of life.

In Hubert Humphrey's time, that test was largely defined by success in the implementation of transformative and historic civil rights laws and the Great Society programs. We succeeded, in part, because of leadership in Washington. But we also succeeded, as Dr. Berwick reminds us, because of the inspiration and organizational skill offered by Dr. Martin Luther King Jr., Ralph Abernathy, John Lewis, and thousands of others like them, in Selma, in Montgomery, and in places like those all over the country.

In meeting the moral test of our day, as we consider our own call to action, we cannot wait for today's Hubert Humphreys in Congress alone to lead us. Passing the test of this generation will require that we all be the agents of change. That we all carry the torch.

And though we can be extremely grateful that we have Don Berwick to inspire us, it is now up to each of us to act.

THE MORAL TEST

PLENARY ADDRESS
INSTITUTE FOR HEALTHCARE IMPROVEMENT
23RD ANNUAL NATIONAL FORUM ON QUALITY
IMPROVEMENT IN HEALTH CARE
ORLANDO, FLORIDA, DECEMBER 7, 2011

LET ME BEGIN by thanking the Picker Institute for this honor [the Picker Institute Award for Excellence]. I am touched to be in such good company, and especially for a theme so close to my heart: patient-centered care. And let me also say a word of personal reverence for Harvey Picker. He was a man of grace, vision, and action. He changed forever our understanding about the proper relationship between the people who get care and the people who give it.

And, I need to say a word about Maureen Bisognano. For years, I have known that the luckiest step in my entire professional career was Maureen's joining IHI in 1995. She made IHI into the organization it has become. She is the best colleague I have ever had—bar none. Now I know that that was the second luckiest step. The *new* luckiest step was Maureen's willingness to become IHI's president and CEO. Thanks to her, I can see after this time away, IHI has soared to entirely new heights with stronger patient voice, wider global reach, an Open School that now includes seventy-four thousand students, and a whole new level of presence and gravitas in the global health care scene. Maureen, you are a treasure—a global treasure—and it is an honor to have you as our leader.

It is good to be back. For me, the past sixteen months have been quite an expedition; I feel like Marco Polo. Never having expected it, I journeyed into the world of national policy and politics at the most tumultuous time for both modern American health care and the modern global economy. To keep things in perspective, I also watched grandson number one—Nathaniel—grow to two-and-a-half-years old, and we welcomed grandson number two—Caleb—into the world just eight weeks ago.

The time at CMS [Centers for Medicare & Medicaid Services] has been a privilege. I got the chance to work with thousands of career public servants, and to learn how much these people do for us all, unsung and too often unappreciated. These are the people who translate laws into regulations and regulations into deeds. At CMS these are the people who keep the lights on—they see that providers get paid, they protect the public trust, and they make sure that the most vulnerable people in America get the care they need.

And, I got the chance to help pilot toward harbor the most important health care policy of our time: the Affordable Care Act. It is a majestic law. I learned, though, that a law is only a framework; it's like an architect's sketch. If it's going to help anyone, it has to be transformed into the specifications like regulations and guidance documents. Only then can it become real programs with real resources that reach real people. On my expedition, that, mostly, was what I was doing.

I would have loved to keep at that job longer. But, as you know, the politics of Washington, and especially the politics of the United States Senate, said, "No." But, overall, I don't have an ounce of regret. What I feel is grateful for the chance I had to serve, and for the generous support I felt, including from so many of you.

I want this afternoon to share with you a little of what I learned on the expedition; and what I think it means for you—for all of us. It's a sort of good-news/bad-news situation. The good news: the possibility of change has never been greater—not in my lifetime. The bad news: if it's going to be the right change, the burden is yours.

When I first got the job, my brother, Bob, a retired middle school science teacher and a very wise man, gave me a sign to put on my desk. It read, "How will it help the patient?" That sign was there from the minute I arrived until the minute I left. Maureen gave me the same sort of advice just before I left IHI. I asked her how I could succeed at CMS, and she said, "That's easy; just mention a patient five times a day."

Bob's advice and Maureen's was the best I got—hands down—from anyone else, anywhere else. Remember the patient.

As it turns out, that's not easy in an office just a few hundred yards from the US Capitol Building—just a mile and a half from the White House. Every morning at breakfast, the stewards of national policy and politics rush to scan the *Washington Post* and *Politico* and to wolf down the day's Capitol Hill newsletters and blogs. What they are finding out is what each other says. Which senator has raised an eyebrow? Which lobbyist has cried foul? Which committee is launching which outraged inquiry into which shocking development? In Washington, a day without a shocking development is hardly worth getting up for. And, of course, who is ahead? Always, who is ahead? My son, Dan, when he first knew I was going to Washington, and who had lived there, said to me, "Just remember, Dad, Washington is a city where everyone is trying to get into a room they aren't yet in."

In that self-absorbed culture, the question, "How does it help the patient?," isn't always the first one asked. In fact, it can seem naïve—not the point. And yet, I learned that, in Washington, D.C., just like here, it is exactly the right question. The best public policy and the best public management answer it. This is only Harvey Picker's idea reframed—from patient-centered care to patient-centered policy.

And that leads me to a second big lesson. I can best explain it to you by describing a visit I made in the fall of 2011 to a small rural hospital— Lower Umpqua Hospital in Reedsport, Oregon. I was on a so-called "rural road trip," visiting rural hospitals to learn from them.

At a meeting there, one of the doctors spoke up—Dr. Robert Law— and he captivated me. Dr. Law, I learned, was the Oregon Academy of Family Practice's "Family Physician of the Year" in 1999. And two sentences into his remarks at the meeting, I could see why. He spoke from his heart. He said how deeply he cared about his community, his patients, and his professionalism. He told why he felt lucky to be serving, and how willing he was to try out new ways to meet needs, even while resources get tighter. He said how offended he was by waste in the health care system—even in Reedsport—and how hard he wanted to work to make sure that every single thing done to, for, and with patients and families would actually help them—on their terms, not his. And—most importantly—he asked for help—for a context of policy, payment, and information that, simply put, would help him get his work done with pride and joy. "If things don't change soon," he told me last week, "I am not sure how we can keep going."

Cynicism grips Washington. It grips Washington far too much . . . far too much for a place that could instead remind us continually of the grandeur of democracy. I vividly remember my first trip ever to Washington, D.C. I was twelve years old, and friends took me to the Lincoln Memorial just after sunset. I looked from the statue of Abraham Lincoln, past the reflecting pool and the Washington Monument, to the glowing Capitol building in the distance—the same Capitol that I saw outside my office window every day for the past sixteen months. And, twelve years old, I cried in awe and admiration for—what shall I call it?—majesty.

Two weeks ago, Congress's approval rating fell to an all-time low: 9 percent.

How did that happen? It happens when the cynics are winning. In a city where everyone wishes to be in a room they are not yet in, it is easy to see everyone as on the make, everyone maneuvering, everyone with elbows sharpened. It becomes too easy to lose hope and confidence, and to forget what can be noble in human nature.

When the lens through which one sees the world magnifies combat, dissembling, and greed, then trust decays and those who deserve to be trusted feel bad—misunderstood, confused, and impeded in their good works.

Dr. Robert Law is not cynical, and he is not on the make. He is dedicated to a life of service to a community he loves, and in which he raised his own three children—Alison, Brian, and Duncan. The job of public servants is to serve him so that he can better serve others. He needs help, resources, encouragement, voice, and respect. His promise—what he can offer our nation—has nothing to do with preventing fraud, holding his feet to the fire, or audits, and it has little to do with payment for performance, public measurement, incentives, or accountability. He is a good person who needs dignified assistance to do good work . . . and he is legion. He can be the future. He, in fact, can and will rescue us, if we will help him help us.

If lesson one for me is, "Remember the patient," then lesson two is this: "Help those who help others." Those thoughts—not the negativity— guided my work in D.C., and they made my time there meaningful.

They are reminders of what is truly important; not the noise, but simply this: to help the people who need our help the most.

Inscribed on the wall of the great hall at the entrance to the Hubert Humphrey Building, the HHS headquarters in Washington where my office was, is a quotation from Senator Humphrey at the building's dedication ceremony on November 4, 1977. It says, "The moral test of government is how it treats those who are in the dawn of life, the children; those who are in the twilight of life, the aged; and those in the shadows of life, the sick, the needy and the handicapped."

I believe that. Indeed, I think that Senator Humphrey described the moral test, not just of government, but of a nation. This is a time of great strain in America; uncertainty abounds. With uncertainty comes fear, and with fear comes withdrawal. We can climb into our bunkers, each separately, and bar the door. But, remember, millions of Americans don't have a bunker to climb into—they have no place to hide. For many of them, indeed, the crisis of economic security that we all dread now is no crisis at all—it is their status quo. The Great Recession is just their normal life.

The rate of poverty in this country is rising. Over one hundred million Americans—nearly one in every three of us—are in poverty or near-poverty today—seventeen million of them children. I will tell you—state by state, community by community, and in the halls of Washington, itself—the security of the poor—their ability to find the health care they need, and the food, and the housing, and the jobs, and the schools—all of it, hangs by a thread. The politics of poverty have never been power politics in America, for the simple reason that the poor don't vote and the children don't vote and the sickest among us don't vote. And, if those who do vote do not assert firmly that Senator Humphrey was right, and if we do not insist on a government that passes the moral test—the thread will break, and shame on us if it does. Cynicism diverts energy from the great moral test. It toys with deception, and deception destroys. Let me give you an example: the outrageous rhetoric about "death panels"—the claim, nonsense, fabricated out of nothing but fear and lies, that some plot is afoot to, literally, kill patients under the guise of end-of-life care. That is hogwash. It is purveyed by cynics; it employs deception; and it destroys hope. It is beyond cruelty to have subjected our elders, especially, to groundless fear in the pure service of political agendas.

The truth, of course, is that there are no "death panels" here, and there never have been. The *truth* is that, as our society has aged and as we have learned to care well for the chronically ill, many of us face years in the twilight of our lives when our health fades and our need for help grows and changes. Luckily, palliative care—care that brings comfort, company, and spiritual and emotional support to people with advanced illness and their families—has grown at its best into a fine art and a better science. The principle is simple: that we can and should offer people the very best of care at all stages of their lives, including the twilight. The truth is, furthermore, that patient-centered care demands that the ways in which a person is cared for ought always to be under his or her control. The patient is the boss; we are the servants. They, not others, should direct their own care, and the doctors, nurses, and hospitals should know and honor what the patient wants. Some of us want to be guaranteed that, no matter how sick or close to death we are, every single machine, drug, and device that could help us live even a moment longer should be used; and that is, therefore, exactly what they should have. And, others of us want not to spend our final days in an intensive care unit, attached to machines, but rather, say, to be at home, in our own bed surrounded by our loved ones in a familiar place, but still receiving world-class treatment for pain and complications; then that is, therefore, exactly what *they* should have. It is one of the great and needless tragedies of this stormy time in health care that the "death panel" rhetoric has denied patients the care that they want, denied caregivers the information they need to give that care, and denied our nation access to a mature, open, informed, and balanced discussion of the challenge of advanced illness and the commitment to individual dignity. It is a travesty.

If you really want to talk about "death panels," let's think about what happens if we cut back programs of needed, life-saving care for Medicaid beneficiaries and other poor people in America. What happens in a nation willing to say to a senior citizen of marginal income, "I am sorry you cannot afford your medicines, but you are on your own"? What happens if we choose to defund our nation's investments in preventive medicine and community health, condemning a generation to avoidable risks and unseen toxins? Maybe a real death panel is a group of people who tell health care insurers that it is okay to take insurance away from people because they are sick or are at risk for becoming sick. Enough of "death panels"! How about all of us—all of us in America—becoming a *life* panel, unwilling to rest easy, in what is still the wealthiest nation on Earth, while a single person within our borders lacks access to the health care they need as a basic human right? Now, *that* is a conversation worth having.

And, while we are at it, what about "rationing"? The distorted and demagogic use of that term is another travesty in our public debate. In some way, the whole idea of improvement—the whole, wonderful idea that brings us—thousands—together this very afternoon is that rationing—denying care to anyone who needs it—is not necessary. That is, it is not necessary if, and only if, we work tirelessly and always to improve the way we try to meet that need.

The true rationers are those who impede improvement, who stand in the way of change, and who thereby force choices that we can avoid through better care. It boggles my mind that the same people who cry "foul" about rationing an instant later argue to reduce health care benefits for the needy, to defund crucial programs of care and prevention, and to shift thousands of dollars of annual costs to people—elders, the poor, the disabled—who are least able to bear them. When the seventeen million American children who live in poverty cannot get the immunizations and blood tests they need, *that* is rationing. When disabled Americans lack the help to keep them out of institutions and in their homes and living independently, *that* is rationing. When tens of thousands of Medicaid beneficiaries are thrown out of coverage, and when millions of seniors are threatened with the withdrawal of preventive care or cannot afford their medications, and when every single one of us lives under the sword of Damocles that, if we get sick, we lose health insurance, *that* is rationing. And it is beneath us as a great nation to allow that to happen.

And that brings me to the opportunity we now have and a duty. A moral duty: to rescue American health care the only way it can be rescued—by improving it.

I have never seen, nor had I dared hope to see, an era in American health care when that is more possible than this very moment. The signs are everywhere. In the past two years, major hospital systems are asking at last how they can coordinate care. Specialty societies are coalescing around plans for more evidence-based care, the use of clinical registries, serious recertification, and reduction of overuse of unhelpful care. The patient safety movement is maturing, with numerous national efforts to bring excellence to scale, including the billion-dollar Partnership for Patients that we launched in HHS. Insurers are experimenting with much more integrated payment models, of which accountable care organizations are only one breed. Transparency is, I believe and hope, about to leap forward. Patients' and consumers' groups are more active and more sophisticated, and they are gaining the footholds they need in governance. Employer groups and labor unions are uniting in their demands. And states are on the move—states like Oregon, Arkansas, and Massachusetts—where courageous and visionary governors—like John Kitzhaber, Mike Beebe, and Deval Patrick—are catalyzing transformation.

And, though no sane person would have wished on us the most serious economic crisis since the Great Depression, the global downturn has added tons to the pressure for change. We are headed for a cliff, and we need to change course. And that means health care needs to change course.

To be clear, we have not changed course yet. Not enough. Not hardly. All the unfreezing has not yet moved health care into its new and needed state. In truth, we have only been getting ready. The Affordable Care Act helps, but a law is not change—it sets the table for change. A constitutional provision for a free press does nothing until the presses start to turn. And a law that provides support for seamless, coordinated care has done nothing until some person who needs it gets it.

This is the threshold we have now come to, but not yet crossed: the threshold from the care we have to the care we need.

We can do this . . . we who give care. And nobody else can. The buck has stopped. The federal framework is set by the Affordable Care Act and important prior laws, such as the HITECH Act, and, quite frankly, we can't expect any bold statutory movement with a divided Congress within the next year or more. The buck has stopped; it has stopped with you.

Now comes the choice. To change, or not to change.

It is not possible to claim that we do not know what to do. We have the templates.

If you doubt it, visit the brilliant Nuka care system at Southcentral Foundation in Anchorage, which just won the Baldrige Award. I visited in October. Thoroughly integrated teams of caregivers—physicians, advanced practice nurses, behavioral health specialists, nutritionists, and more—occupy open physical pods in line-of-sight contact with each other all day long, weaving a net of help and partnership with Alaska Native patients and families. The results: 60 percent fewer emergency and urgent care visits, 50 percent fewer hospitalizations, and 40 percent less use of specialists, along with staff turnover one-fifth as frequent as before the new care.

If you doubt that we know what to do, visit Denver Health or Theda-Care or Virginia Mason, and see the Toyota principles of Lean production learned, mastered, adapted, and deployed through entire systems and into the skills and psyches of entire workforces. The result, over $100 million in savings at Denver Health, while vastly improving the experience and outcomes of patients.

If you doubt that we know what to do, contact George Halvorson at Kaiser Permanente and ask him how they have reduced sepsis mortality— sepsis is the cause of death in 24 percent of seniors who die in California hospitals. Kaiser Permanente has driven down sepsis mortality by nearly half—to 11 percent in less than three years.

Let me put it simply: in this room, with the successes already in hand among you here, you collectively have enough knowledge to rescue American health care—hands down. Better care, better health, and lower cost through improvement right here. In this room.

The only question left is, will you do it?

When we entered the world of health care improvement as our life's work, we didn't ask for the burden we now bear. We did not ask to be responsible for rescuing health care.

But, here we are, and, as intimidating as the fact may be, that burden is ours. Our nation is at a crossroads. The care we have simply cannot be sustained. It will not work for health care to chew ever more deeply into our common purse. If it does, our schools will fail, our roads will fail, our competitiveness will fail. Wages will continue to lag, and, paradoxically, so will our health.

The choice is stark: chop or improve. If we permit chopping, I assure you that the chopping block will get very full—first with cuts to the most voiceless and poorest of us, but, soon after, to more and more of us. Fewer health insurance benefits, declining access, more out-of-pocket burdens, and growing delays. If we don't improve, the cynics win.

That's what passes the buck to us. If improvement is the plan, then we own the plan. Government can't do it. Payers can't do it. Regulators can't do it. Only the people who give the care can improve the care.

What's the strategy? Let me show you one. I owe much of this to my friend and colleague, Andy Hackbarth, who has been collaborating with Joe McCannon, others, and me for much of the year to develop a set of lenses clear enough to let us see the pathway to success.

We began with work far from health care—the work of a Princeton economist and environmental expert named Robert Socolow. Professor Socolow published an important article in 2004 in *Science* magazine, trying to answer a very important question: "What is the way to slow the rate of atmospheric carbon production enough to avert catastrophic carbon levels in the future?"

Here is his answer: "There is no way." That is, there is no *single* way to do it. Automobile emission control can't do it. Solar power can't do it. Conservation can't do it. The only way we can do it is to do, not one thing, but everything. When I read Socolow's article, I thought instantly of Göran Henrik's answer to me when I asked him a few years ago how Jönköping County in Sweden was achieving such pace-setting results in total health system performance. Göran said, "Here's the secret: We do everything."

"Do everything"—that's Socolow's answer to the global warming problem. Luckily, nothing more than everything is necessary, and, unluckily, nothing less than everything is sufficient. Socolow diagrammed "everything" as what he called "wedges."

The wedges—Socolow proposes fifteen of them—fifteen changes that affect carbon output—fill what Socolow calls the "sustainability triangle." The wedges framework looks a lot like a strategic plan, or at least a system of strategic goals, whose cumulative effect—all together—is a sustainable level of carbon, so that we don't cook Planet Earth.

Solving the health care crisis has wedges, too. We don't have as crystal clear a target—a sustainability level that works for total US health care spending—but for sure our "business as usual" line isn't it. Pay on that line over time, and schools suffer, roads suffer, museums suffer, and private consumption suffers because, as Tom Nolan said years ago, "It's our money." It is all wages.

Now, I probably owe you an apology for talking about costs. I know that, among the important dimensions of quality—safety, effectiveness, patient-centered care, timeliness, efficiency, and equity—I am not sure any of us would have chosen efficiency—the reduction of waste—as our favorite. It's not my favorite. Nonetheless, it is the quality dimension of our time. I would go so far as to say that, for the next three to five years at least, the credibility and leverage of the quality movement will rise or fall on its success in reducing the cost of health care—and, harder, returning that money to other uses—while improving patient experience. Value improvement won't be enough; it will take cost reduction to capture the flag. Otherwise, cutting wins.

But, I am not going to apologize. That's because if you are a student of Lean thinking or quality, itself—if you have taken the time to study the work of Noriaki Kano, or Jim Womack, or Taichi Ohno, or Dr. Deming, you know that great leverage in cost reduction comes directly—powerfully—exactly from focusing on meeting the needs of the person you serve. *Waste* is actually just a word that means "not helpful." So, that initial wave of reaction—"Who wants to work on efficiency?"—is actually off the mark. In very large measure, improving care and reducing waste are one and the same thing.

How much cost reduction? Well, if we look to Europe for ideas, then a target of, say, 12 percent of our GDP, far below our current 17 percent, would look plausible. If you want to stay at home for signals, find the lowest cost quartile of American health care economies—hospital referral regions, or HRRs—and we'd be somewhere in the neighborhood of 15 percent of GDP. Or maybe that looks tough, and you'd be more comfortable if health care began to behave just as well as, but no better than, the rest of the economy—that is, rising in sync with the GDP, itself, and just staying where it is—17 percent or so.

The point is, with costs rising a great deal faster than that, no matter what your goal is, you've got a sustainability triangle to fill—the growing, cumulative difference between unsustainable "business as usual" costs and the sustainable ones.

The social imperative for reducing health care costs is enormous. And, to meet that enormous need, I suggest, just as with the environmental triangle, for the health care cost triangle, nothing works. Only everything works. It's all or none, or we head straight on and over the cliff.

Andy Hackbarth and I took a stab at defining the "wedges" for health care costs. These are the names of the forms of waste whose removal from the system both helps patients thrive and reduces the cost of care. We found six wedges, for starters, and we estimated their size.

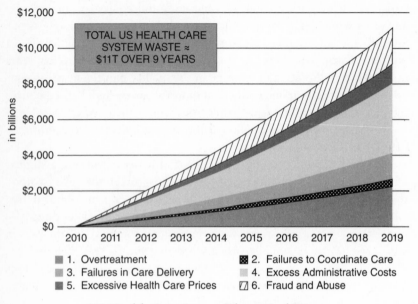

US Health Care System Theoretical Waste
(Aggregate Waste 2011–2019)

1. *Overtreatment:* The waste that comes from subjecting people to care that cannot possibly help them—care rooted in outmoded habits, supply-driven behaviors, and ignoring science.

2. *Failures of Coordination:* The waste that comes when people— especially people with chronic illness—fall through the slats. They get lost, forgotten, confused. The result: complications, decays in functional status, hospital readmissions, and dependency.

3. *Failures of Reliability:* The waste that comes with poor execution of what we know to do. The result: safety hazards and worse outcomes.

4. *Administrative Complexity:* The waste that comes when we create our own rules that force people to do things that make no sense—

that converts valuable nursing time into meaningless charting rituals
or limited physician time into nonsensical and complex billing
procedures.

5. *Pricing Failures:* The waste that comes as prices migrate far from
   the actual costs of production plus fair profits.

6. *Fraud and Abuse:* The waste that comes as thieves steal what is not
   theirs, and also from the blunt procedures of inspection and regulation that infect everyone because of the misbehaviors of a very few.

We have estimated how big this waste is—from both the perspective
of the federal payers—Medicare and Medicaid—and for all payers.
Research and analytic literature contain a very wide range of estimates,
but, at the median, the total annual level of waste in just these six categories (and I am sure there are more) exceeds $1 trillion every year—perhaps
a third of our total cost of production.

This is our task—our unwelcome task—if we are to help save health
care from the cliff. To reduce costs, by reducing waste, at scale, everywhere, now.

I recommend five principles to guide that investment:

1. *Put the patient first.* Every single deed—every single change—
   should protect, preserve, and enhance the well-being of the people
   who need us. That way—and only that way—we will know waste
   when we see it.

2. Among patients, *put the poor and disadvantaged first*—those in the
   beginning, the end, and the shadows of life. Let us meet the moral
   test.

3. *Start at scale.* There is no more time left for timidity. Pilots will
   not suffice. The time has come, to use Göran Henrik's scary
   phrase, to do everything. In basketball, they call it "flooding the
   zone." It's time to flood the Triple Aim zone.

4. *Return the money.* This is the hardest principle of them all.
   Success will not be in our hands unless and until the parties
   burdened by health care costs feel that burden to be lighter. It is
   crucial that the employers and wage earners and unions and states
   and taxpayers—those who actually pay the health care bill—see
   that bill fall.

5. *Act locally.* The moment has arrived for every state, community,
   organization, and profession to act. We need mobilization—
   nothing less.

One evening shortly before I left Washington, I visited the Lincoln Memorial again—standing at the same spot that I had stood at as a twelve-year-old boy fifty-three years ago. The majesty was still there—the visage of Lincoln, the reach of the Washington Monument, the glow of the Capitol dome. It was still unbearably beautiful. Still majestic.

But, there was one change. Chiseled in the very stone where I was standing is now the name of Dr. Martin Luther King and the date—August 28, 1963—when he gave his immortal "I have a dream" speech.

When I first stood at that spot, the Montgomery bus boycott was only three years in the past, and Dr. King's speech lay five years in the future. Rachel Carson's book, *Silent Spring*, was four years in the future. And it would be six years before the phrase, "women's liberation," would first be used in America.

I thought, standing there, of something I once heard Dr. Joseph Juran say: "The pace of change is majestic." And I mused about *that* majesty, and its nature.

It occurred to me that the true majesty lay not just in the words—not just in the call—but also in the long and innumerable connections between the ideas that stir us—the dreams—and the millions and millions of tiny, local actions that are the change, at last. A dream of civil rights becomes real only when one black child and one white child take one cooling drink from the same water fountain or use the same bathroom or dine together before the movie they enjoy together. An environmental movement becomes real only when one family places one recycle bin under one sink or turns off one unneeded light out of respect for an unborn generation. Women's rights are not real until one woman's paycheck stub reads the same as one man's, and until my daughter really can be anything she wants to be. The majesty is in the words, but the angel is in the details.

And that is where you come in. Here is the lesson I bring you from seventeen months in Washington, D.C. Your time has come. You are on the cusp of history—you, not Washington, are the bridge between the dream and the reality—or else there will be no bridge. Our quest—for health care that is just, safe, infinitely humane, and that takes only its fair share of our wealth—our quest may not be as magnificent as the quest for human rights or for a sustainable Earth, but it is immensely worthy. You stand, though you did not choose it, at the crossroads of momentous change—at the threshold of majesty. And—frightened, fortunate, or both—you now have a chance to make what is possible real.

FURTHER READING

Berwick DM, Hackbarth AD. Eliminating waste in US health care. *JAMA*.
    2012 Apr 11;307(14):1513–1516.
Pacala S, Socolow R. Stabilization wedges: Solving the climate problem for the
    next 50 years with current technologies. *Science*. 2004;305(5686):
    968–972.

Chapter 14

NEW HEALTH SYSTEM—NEW PROFESSIONALISM

COMMENTARY

James Reason

WHAT WAS A horrible episode for Don (and none too pleasant for Baby Gray), a time of anguish and regret, has been transformed into a huge benefit for health care and for humankind in general. Like other great healers, Don learned from his very understandable mistake. In that regard, consider the "Could-it-have-happened-to-me?" test. I'm sure if this were applied to other pediatric residents and even to more senior doctors, the answer would be in the affirmative.

For the greater part of the ensuing thirty years, Don devoted himself to patient safety. This path led to the establishment of the enormously influential Institute for Healthcare Improvement (IHI). Among its many achievements was the 100,000 Lives Campaign, launched in December 2004, a national initiative whose goal was to reduce unnecessary hospital deaths by one hundred thousand within eighteen months. The Campaign recommended that US hospitals introduce six best-practice interventions:

Deployment of Rapid Response Teams: Emergency
teams comprising clinicians who bring critical care
expertise to the patient's bedside or wherever it is
required

*Delivery of Reliable Evidence-Based Care for Acute
Myocardial Infarction:* Measures to prevent deaths from
heart attack

Prevention of Adverse Drug Events: Achieved by
implementing medication reconciliation

Prevention of Central Line Infections: Using a series of
independent, scientifically grounded steps called the
Central Line Bundle

Prevention of Surgical Site Infections: Achieved by
delivering the correct perioperative antibiotics at the
right time, and

Prevention of Ventilator-Associated Pneumonia:
Achieved by correctly implementing the Ventilator
Bundle

By early 2006, 76 percent of the 3,037 hospitals involved
had submitted mortality data, and the Campaign estimated
that the total number of lives saved would be 58,133. When
this was extrapolated to the middle of 2006, it gave a
projection of 74,573 lives saved. When the likely
improvements associated with quality interventions were
factored in, the estimated number of lives saved in
participating hospitals came to 86,482. The current estimates
are well over 100,000. This is a remarkable achievement—
more than adequate payback for Baby Gray's near miss.

In this commentary, Don has invited me to express my own
views of the safety of health care. Notwithstanding the
pioneering work of the anesthetists and the Harvard Medical
Practice Study, it is convenient to date the current widespread
concern with patient safety from the beginning of the
millennium. That was when the enormously influential US
Institute of Medicine report, *Crossing the Quality Chasm*,
galvanized the attention of a broader health care readership.
This report was quickly followed by a series of high-level
publications from a number of countries. Unlike other
hazardous domains, there was no widely publicized "Big

Bang" event that engendered this concern; just these widely read national reports that detailed the huge costs of adverse events in health care, both in terms of lives lost and money expended. It was clear that the problem was huge and that it existed everywhere.

There is nothing specifically medical about medical errors; the only thing uniquely medical about them is the context in which they occur. Health care professionals—just like the rest of us—are human and so are fallible.

A paradox lies at the heart of the patient safety problem; it has two contradictory elements. First, health care training, particularly that of doctors, is predicated on a belief in trained perfectibility. After a very long, arduous, and expensive education, you are expected to get it right. As a consequence, medical errors are marginalized and stigmatized. Errors, by and large, are equated to incompetence. A consequence is that, unlike in aviation, there has been little or no tradition of reporting and learning from errors.

The second part of the paradox is that health care activities are among the most error-provoking on the planet. This is true for a variety of reasons: a huge diversity of activities and equipment; hands-on work with limited safeguards; vulnerable and easily harmed patients; local event investigation, with little or no widespread learning; and one-to-one or few-to-one deliveries, both of which increase the chances of damaging errors.

I have had the great pleasure of working with Don Berwick over the past decade, but usually in faraway places. Following his period as administrator of the Centers for Medicare & Medicaid Services (CMS), his proven patient safety prowess has brought him, for me at least, closer to home. He has been chosen by our prime minister, David Cameron, to head a national advisory group on the safety of patients in England. This followed a public inquiry report of the shocking conditions that existed in one of our National Health System's hospitals. I am delighted to say that I am a part of this advisory group.

The patient safety movement, more than most, needs effective and wholly committed leadership. Fortunately, we have Don Berwick.

NEW HEALTH
SYSTEM—NEW
PROFESSIONALISM

GAY LECTURE, HARVARD MEDICAL SCHOOL
BOSTON, MASSACHUSETTS, APRIL 14, 2012

IT WAS 1974. I was midway in my first year of pediatric residency, after an initial year in internal medicine, and on my second rotation in neonatal intensive care. My first was at Boston Children's Hospital; this one was at the old Boston Lying-in Hospital, across the street.

It was 3 o'clock in the morning. The nurse had awoken me from a fitful sleep to do the next exchange transfusion for baby—let's call him "Baby Gray."

Many of you here may have no idea of what an exchange transfusion is or what it involves. It was a mainstay of neonatal intensive care in those days, but now it's almost never necessary. It was the treatment for *erythroblastosis fetalis*, the life-threatening hemolytic anemia that came from incompatibility between a baby's blood type and its mother's— often an Rh factor incompatibility. An Rh-positive baby developed inside an Rh-negative mother who had previously borne an Rh-positive baby. Sensitized by peripartum exposure to the alien antigen in the former baby's blood, the mother carried anti-Rh antibodies, which attacked the red cells of the new baby, causing hemolysis, anemia, and, potentially, death.

The treatment kept many a pediatric resident awake nights; it was called "exchange transfusion." The idea was to substitute Rh-negative blood for the baby's own in the newborn period, removing both the

226

vulnerable cells and the mother's circulating antibodies—long enough for the residual antibodies in the baby's bloodstream to break down. It saved lives.

It was a mechanical thing. Canulate the baby's umbilical vein with a sterile catheter. Get Rh negative—O negative—from the blood bank, and hook up a three-way stopcock and a syringe. Draw, say, 10 ccs from the baby, turn the stopcock, evacuate the blood into a waste basket, turn the stopcock, draw down 10 ccs of blood from the bank bag, turn the stopcock, and slowly push the new blood into the baby. Do that, say, fifty times; then go get some rest. And then, four hours later, do it again. I think about this every time my automobile mechanic flushes my radiator for the new season.

I walked, bleary, to Baby Gray's incubator, took the bag of blood from the nurse, connected the stopcock gear, and started. This was my first exchange transfusion at the Lying-in Hospital; I had done a half dozen or so at Children's.

Something was wrong. I knew it after just a few of those boring cycles. The syringe felt sticky, and I wondered if I was pushing too hard. But I went on. After fifteen or twenty minutes, the vague feeling had become an alarming one. Baby Gray looked gray. He was squirming, mottled, and his heart rate had risen—a lot. I was perplexed, ordered some STAT tests, and asked the nurse to page the neonatal fellow, who was asleep at home in Newton, as they did in those days, seven miles away. I stopped the transfusion, sweated, and tried, without success, to figure out what Baby Gray's problem was.

Twenty minutes later, the fellow walked in, and, just then, the lab tech brought me the STAT results. I couldn't believe what I saw. Baby Gray's hematocrit was 90 percent—his blood was as thick as molasses—almost no plasma at all, just red cells. That's why he looked so bad—and he did look bad.

I clutched. For the life of me, I could not figure out why the baby had gone bad. And then, the fellow saw it. Dangling down from the bag of bank blood I had tapped for the exchange was a second bag, full of pure, clear plasma, connected by a tube to the bag I had canulated.

That was the answer. The blood bank had centrifuged this blood when it was collected, and stored it as two separate but connected bags—one with packed red blood cells, and one with fresh serum. It was logical. If you needed just packed cells, they were ready. If you needed plasma, it was ready, too. And, if you needed whole blood, as I did for the exchange transfusion, all you had to do was to remix the two bags and—*voila!*—whole blood.

I did not do that. I did not see that. I did not know that. I was trans-fusing Baby Gray with packed red blood cells. And he was dying from that mistake.

The fellow whipped into action. He started a mini-exchange with the plasma, only, ordered whole blood from the blood bank, and, as soon as it arrived, did a new exchange with the whole blood.

Baby Gray lived. I think he lived. He went into acute renal failure that night, but his blood pressure and pulse normalized. Gradually over the next few days, as his kidneys were washed by the new, good blood, they opened up, and his renal function normalized. I left the hospital before Baby Gray did—on to my next rotation, back at Children's Hospital.

But I remember that night now—right now—with all of the tension and fear and guilt and self-loathing that I felt at that moment. I remember—I feel—my thought: "How could I have been so stupid? How could I have been so stupid?"

Not that the fellow said that to me. He did not. He put his arm over my shoulder, and said, "Don't feel so bad; this could have happened to anybody." Maybe he thought that. I don't know. I didn't think that. It hadn't happened to anybody. It had happened to me, and to my patient. And how, in God's name, *how* could I have been so stupid?

Now, I would like you to guess something. Guess—what did I do? Not, what did I *feel*, but what did I *do*?

One answer you cannot offer; it's too obvious. Too easy. One thing I did was cry. Not on the spot, but a half-hour later, back in the on-call room, alone, mortified, terrified. Of course, I cried.

I don't mean that. I mean, what did I do the next day? In follow-up? The day after? The week after? The year after?

I wish I could tell you that the answer is this: the next day—I wish I could say—I went to see the head of the Boston Lying-in Blood Bank, and told him or her what I had done. That, at the Children's Hospital Blood Bank, across the street, they did not centrifuge blood in advance, separately storing cell and plasma. They did that when it was needed; they stored the blood there as whole blood. I was tired, and I missed the obvious. And that, maybe, just maybe, a standardized procedure would be a bit safer.

I wish I could say that I called up the head of the residency training program, the guy who would eventually be writing my letters of recom-mendation and launching me on my future trajectory, and suggest that some orientation to different processes when a resident switches sites would be helpful.

I wish I could say that, when all of my fellow residents got together for grand rounds or a pizza party that week, I shushed them down and said, "Hey, everybody, listen up. I almost killed a baby last night, and I'd like to tell you how so that it won't happen to you, at least not that way."

But, did I do that? No, of course not. The right answer to my question, "What did I do?" is, simply, "Nothing." I did nothing. The secret of my failure—the secret of my stupidity—the secret of my sin—stayed quietly—no, painfully—in my heart, and in the gentle, encouraging mind of the fellow.

I did nothing because, if it had occurred to me to do something, which it did not, I would have been absolutely sure that, no matter what the blood bank head, or residency head, or my fellow interns might say—no matter how much they would smile, pat me on my back, and say, "It could have happened to anyone"—they would know, and they would think, and they would say to each other, when I was not there, exactly what I knew and thought and was saying to myself, then, as I will for the rest of my life: "How could he have been so stupid?"

I am no expert in ethics. As an amateur, I imagine that mostly it's a topic about individuals. A person is ethical, or not. Are communities ethical? Are organizations ethical? Systems?

I have been for thirty years a student of quality. It fascinates me to ask, "Where does performance come from? How does improvement occur?" *Quality* is, in this regard, a nearly useless word. It is overbroad. It makes more sense to me to think beneath it—to closer, clearer thinking about what, after all, is good. What do we want? Whom do we serve? And what do they want? We do better, by definition, when we better meet the need we intend to serve.

One thing is for sure: Baby Gray wanted not to nearly die. He was busy entering life. What happened to him—what I did to him—was, by any name, bad. It was a quality defect. A thing gone wrong. Today, we would call it a medical error, an adverse event, or a patient safety problem.

As an amateur ethicist, it seems to me it was unethical to allow Baby Gray to be injured. And, I would add, crucially, it would be doubly unethical ever—ever—to allow another baby to be injured by the same cause—there, across the street, or anywhere at all.

So, with respect to Baby Gray, who violated the ethics? Was it I? Tired, careless, stupid I? Scarred, scared I?

Maybe to find out the answer, we need to become a little more scientific about the investigation. If we know the cause, maybe we can fix the blame.

The science of safety is vast. The study of things gone wrong—failures—is now a century old, and has had serious, pregnant formulations for at least half a century. Among the most powerful contributors, and I hope you know his name, is Professor James Reason of Manchester University. He wrote a key book called *Human Error*, which still stands, thirty years after its first publication, as the best of its kind.

Jim Reason invented the so-called Swiss cheese model of errors. He sees the world of causation as a cauldron of bubbles he calls "latent errors," factors that can lead to defect, but that usually do not line up. He says they are like holes in Swiss cheese; usually not lined up. One error occurs, but it is quickly trapped and its effect mitigated by some other resilience in the system. The young, tired resident—okay, the *stupid* resident—does not see the dangling bag of plasma, but the alert nurse does and stops him in time. Or, the young, tired, stupid resident would have missed the set-up, but the blood bank, knowing this is an exchange transfusion, reconstitutes the whole blood before it gets to the floor.

Harm happens—errors become completed—says Reason, when the latent causes, randomly swirling in the ether of our lives and work, happen—just happen—to line up, like the holes in that occasional block of Swiss cheese.

So, the blood bank procedures vary from place to place (latent cause), and Don is groggy from no sleep (latent cause), and the night nurse is new and hasn't assisted an exchange transfusion before (latent cause), and plasma is clear in a clear bag and hard to see at night (latent cause), and no one who has ever done an exchange in that hospital is within seven miles of Baby Gray (latent cause), and . . . and . . . and . . . And the holes line up, and Baby Gray is right there, on the sharp end of the knitting needle.

What, in God's name, are the ethics of that?

I propose two answers, and I think that they are crucial to our mission, to our pride, to our patients, and, just maybe, to the future of health care as a whole.

I propose that the ethics of quality—safety—performance—goodness—reside in two loci, and must be named and owned there. Neither alone is sufficient; both together are sufficient.

First, the ethics of quality lie in the professions—or should. The largest lapse in what we should call ethics in my story, I now believe, is not the damage done to Baby Gray, but in the silence that followed. That I did not speak up; nor did my fellow, nor did a nurse. In our silent, frightened, helpless conspiracy of nonaction, these inactions made it finitely and unacceptably possible that the same injury could happen again to another baby, another time, maybe in another place.

And, not insignificantly, there was another silence. Baby Gray's family never knew. I didn't tell them; I know that. And I suspect very strongly that neither the fellow nor the attending nor the nurse—no one—told the family the truth, the whole truth. "There is a little problem," they maybe said. "He had a bad reaction to a transfusion . . . He'll be okay, we're quite confident." I am quite sure that no one was particularly interested in outing my stupidity, and, if they made a move in that direction, the hospital's lawyers would have shushed them pretty fast.

How, if we are healers, can we conscience the fact that we do not act to prevent harm when we know the cause?

That's a high-minded question. It might even make me look, not just stupid, but unethical. But, of course, there is a vicious trap in that high-minded question. It goes back to me—the next day—age twenty-seven and looking ahead into a career of unknown trajectory and risk. Can it really be expected of me that I will, suicidally, confess my own stupid, nearly lethal incompetence in the vague hope that someone, somewhere downstream will somehow benefit from my selflessness?

"Yes," you say? Or, is it, "No"?

I say, "It depends." And that leads me to the second, and essential, locus of the ethics of improvement: leaders. Suppose I ask you to imagine—can you imagine?—a context in which that next day, full of the knowledge that I had, and, even, still wracked by guilt, I would nonetheless have brought forth what I knew to people who could do something about it—people who, unlike me, could change the latent causes, close down some bubbles, prevent their future alignment. Could you imagine that I had been told, as a definition of the professional I would some day become, this?

> You are not a superhero, though, caring as you are, you will always
> wish you could be for your patients. You are part of something much
> larger than yourself, and the well-being of your patients, and others'
> patients, depends on your bearing with dignity the burden of saying
> what you see, sharing what you learn, and admitting what goes
> wrong, because, that way, and only that way, can we build stronger
> and stronger and stronger teams and systems of support so that our
> frail, human, fatiguable, trickable, limited minds and bodies can none-
> theless participate in pursuit of what matters—perfection.

Can you imagine a context, and community, in which my good, loving fellow would have said, not, "Don't feel bad; it could have happened to anybody," but rather, "Get some sleep now. Tomorrow, refreshed, we will think together with many others about what happened, why, and how we can together make sure that it will never, ever happen again. You are not alone; and you can help so much."

Now, at the risk of making this harder, I need to carry this one more step. In exploring the ethics of patient safety, I took an easy shot with my story of Baby Gray. I had you at "Hello."

But, remember that "quality," goodness, is multidimensional. Our work meets social needs far beyond safety, alone—social needs for reliability (that our patients will always get the care that helps them, and not the care that does not help them); for equity (that race and ethnicity do not predict health care and outcomes); for patient-centeredness (that, in the final analysis, the patient's preferences control what we do).

And now, in this era, another dimension of social need has come to the foreground: reducing cost. It's not anywhere near as charismatic a pursuit as is the pursuit of safety. If I start to talk about health care costs, I do not have you at "Hello." But, I now believe that, in America at least, the creation and stabilization of a system of care with costs far lower than those of today is an ethical duty. When it comes to cost, no Baby Gray lies helpless at night awaiting the right blood transfusion or the wrong one. But, as health care digs ever deeper into our nation's income, our neighbors' wages, our businesses' vitality, and, most crucially of all, our governments' capacities to do other forms of good, I guarantee to you that millions and millions of people face imminent harm as a result. Our schools totter, our bridges decay, our generosity to the poor wavers, our assistance to the disabled pales, our arts languish, and our standard of living overall hangs in the balance.

Health care costs in America are draining American vitality. And every bit of evidence we have from deep studies of comparative performance— within the United States and among nations—and from detailed explorations of forms of waste—every bit of the evidence suggests that this burden is not necessary. We can have all of the health care we want and need if we cease our concession to waste in the work we do. I have written elsewhere about the dimensions and magnitude of that waste, and will not repeat it here, except to say that I regard it as nearly impossible that less than 20 percent of what we spend in American health care is pure waste—of no value to our mission—and that it is very likely more than one-third.

What does this possibly have to do with ethics and Baby Gray? Everything. That—realizing that—is a transition in self-image and the sense of purpose that I now believe both our professions and our leaders need badly to make.

The next Baby Gray will die unless individual professionals and the leaders who establish the contexts for their work accept the ethical duty to learn from harm and prevent future harm through the continual design and redesign of health care as a system.

And, identically, the harm done to our society by a health care system that wastes beyond its means and rightful share will continue and expand unless and until individual professionals and the leaders who establish the contexts for their work accept the ethical duty to remove waste from the care they give.

This is not easy, and excuses are many. The excuses I had for inaction after Baby Gray were more than enough to render me silent. No one will listen. They will blame me. It is my fault, anyway. Or, it's not my fault; why should I act? I am helpless. I can change nothing.

And hear the excuses for waste. The patients demand it. It's defensive medicine. It's the malpractice system. It's the silly regulators. It's the silly payment system.

The choice is the same: whether and when will a profession and its leaders assume willingly the duty, without excuses, to improve.

Harm to patients is different from wasting scarce social resources. Patient harm is individual, equal opportunity, direct, and attributable. The harm from waste is diffuse, selectively bad for the poor, and indirect— no one wasteful health care deed injures a specific school. Waste, unlike patient injury, is a classical problem of the commons.

Patient safety problems threaten individuals in care. Waste threatens health care as a human right.

Our professions and its leaders have a deep, ethical duty to improve health care in all of its dimensions. Here are the principles we should embrace:

1. Professionals have an affirmative, ever-present duty to participate in and, when possible, lead the improvement of the systems of care in which they work.

2. Health care leaders—by which I mean executives, boards, policy makers, and clinical leaders—have an affirmative, ever-present duty to establish contexts in which professionals' adherence to principle number one is logical, feasible, and supported.

3. No excuses for inaction on principles number one and number two are ethically acceptable.

4. The affirmative duty to improve includes improvement in safety, reliability, cost, and equity of health care. The continual reduction of waste is an ethical obligation.

5. Those who educate professionals and leaders have an affirmative duty to prepare them for the successful discharge of these responsibilities, including the task of securing knowledge of systems and safety sciences in all who assume these roles.

I have nightmares sometimes about that time with Baby Gray. Sometimes I can still feel that syringe stick, and see the baby writhe, and panic in the ignorance, and flash hot through my whole body as I see, again, that bag of plasma, testifying to my guilt.

But, on better nights, I have a different dream. It goes like this—a different next day.

In this dream, my fellow and I go the next day to see both the blood bank head and the residency director. Trained in systems theory, they know the work of Jim Reason and Karl Weick and Donald Norman and Richard Cook. They instantly become curious about system vulnerabilities that they did not yet recognize—holes in the cheese—and they start an improvement team on the spot, asking for a list of good ideas within the week. The ideas cascade as nurses, senior and junior doctors, technicians, and engineers follow a branching tree of the system of causes—variation in processes, fatigue in trainees, communication channels between nurses and doctors, visual cues on equipment and blood supplies—and fully reliable standard practices for blood product use.

They report this to, and are accountable to, the CEOs and CMOs and CNOs of both hospitals, whose explicit aim, under the direction of their boards of trustees, is to become world-class, high-reliability organizations, and who know that Baby Gray's harm was tuition paid for safer and safer care for the future.

I would still wonder, through it all, "How could I be so stupid?" That question might never go away. But it would be a thought a little harder to maintain, a scar a little less deep, when I would notice that my leaders thanked me for my honesty, when I was made cochair of the improvement team to work on blood product safety, and when my brother and sister trainees, at pizza, said to me, "Thanks. That's one less thing we have to worry about now." And that some baby not yet born would not needlessly die somewhere, sometime, because I did not—could not—act.

Chapter 15

TO ISAIAH

COMMENTARY

Mark D. Smith

WHEN THE EXAMINATION room door shuts and it is just a patient and a clinician alone together, it feels natural to rely on our training to salve the wounds we can identify. After all, years of study and training and the process of differential diagnosis focus our attention on the problems of the individual's body and mind. It is also, not inconsequentially, what we get paid for doing. It takes someone like Don Berwick to shake us out of our biomedical mindset and remind us that we are dealing not just with a disease but with a person often buffeted by factors we can't quantify or control. Still, we must help. This is what he eloquently tells us in "To Isaiah."

Though some clinicians try to ignore the world outside their offices, most are pulled to some extent into the fuller lives of their patients; some go there more willingly than others. Don speaks to young physicians about his process of moving from a principally medical focus to a broader social one. My journey was, ironically, the other way around. My initial interest in medicine was not so much because I was interested in physiology or anatomy, but

rather because I was drawn to its broader role in society.

I was drawn to the examination room because it was the place where the cures made possible by biomedical advances meet the complicated, fascinating, and often messy lives where patients live; where genes and disease meet society. And as it happened, I trained at a time and in a place at the beginning of a phenomenon that combined both worlds: San Francisco at the dawning of the HIV epidemic. For me and for many of my generation, HIV work combined exciting, cutting-edge scientific discovery with a quest for social justice, because of the nature of the populations originally affected.

More, perhaps, than most diseases, the HIV epidemic over the past thirty years has been a poster child for this complicated interplay of biomedical science and social tensions, social issues, and indeed, social progress. I like to think that, despite the initial hysteria and bigotry that sometimes characterized the reactions of some people to the epidemic early on, the human face of suffering of gay men that the AIDS epidemic created helped to change society's attitudes toward homosexuality by personalizing them in a way that now has broad ramifications in politics and society. It also helped lead to the "harm reduction" approach to IV drug users.

The AIDS epidemic is a clear example of this complicated interaction of medicine and social issues that is the touchstone of what Don is talking about in his patient Isaiah. Simply put: none of us practices in a vacuum. Isaiah had many, many issues besides his medical condition. Don correctly recognized that some were in Don's control, some in Isaiah's (yes, he was dealt a bad hand, but others have played equally bad hands much better), and some were way beyond their grasp. Despite the current malaise among some physicians about the way the world is changing, doctors and other clinicians still have the great honor and privilege to see into the lives of our patients and influence them for the better. We are also in a position to speak out about the larger societal issues that can have a direct, even overpowering, influence on their health. Because people listen, we should be empowered to speak, whether we came to medicine from our love of science or our desire to improve society.

Don's story is, in a way, the story of one person's journey from the biomedical to the social. My story was the opposite: from the social to the biomedical. In the end, many practitioners will have some admixture of them both. Isaiah's life—and death—shows that both are integral to healing; one cannot cure what ails our patients without the other.

TO ISAIAH

HARVARD MEDICAL SCHOOL AND HARVARD
SCHOOL OF DENTAL MEDICINE CLASS DAY ADDRESS
CAMBRIDGE, MASSACHUSETTS, MAY 24, 2012

THANK YOU FOR letting me share this glorious day with you and your loved ones. Feel good. Feel proud. You've earned it.

In preparation for today, I asked your dean of students what she thinks is on your mind. So, she asked you. The word you used—many of you—was this one: *worried*. You're worried about the constant change around you, uncertain about the future of medicine and dentistry. Worried about whether you can make a decent living. You've boarded a boat, and you don't know where it's going.

I can reassure you. You've made a good choice—a spectacularly good choice. The career you've chosen is going to give you many moments of poetry. My favorite is the moment when the door closes—the click of the catch that leaves you and the patient together in the privacy—the sanctity—of the helping relationship. Doors will open too. You'll find ways to contribute to progress that you cannot possibly anticipate now, any more than I could have dreamed of standing here when I was sitting where you are forty years ago.

But look, I won't lie; I'm worried too. I went to Washington to lead the Centers for Medicare & Medicaid Services, full of hope for our nation's long-overdue journey toward making health care a human right here, at last. In lots of ways, I wasn't disappointed. I often saw good government and the grandeur of democracy—both alive, even if not at the moment entirely well.

Note: This speech was published subsequently by the *Journal of the American Medical Association*, as "A Piece of My Mind: To Isaiah." Berwick, D. M. A piece of my mind: To Isaiah. *Journal of the American Medical Association*. 2012, Jun 27;307(24):2597–2599.

But, like you, I also found much that I could not control—a context torn apart by antagonisms—too many people in leadership, from whom we ought to be able to expect more, willing to bend the truth and rewrite facts for their own convenience. I heard irresponsible, cruel, baseless rhetoric about death panels silence mature, compassionate, scientific inquiry into the care we all need and want in the last stages of our lives. I heard meaningless, cynical accusations about rationing repeated over and over again by the same people who then unsheathed their knives to cut Medicaid. I watched fear grow on both sides of the political aisle— fear of authentic questions, fear of reasoned debate, and fear of tomorrow morning's headlines—fear that stifled the respectful, civil, shared inquiry upon which the health of democracy depends.

And so, Harvard School of Dental Medicine and Harvard Medical School Class of 2012, I'm worried, too. I, too, wonder where this boat is going.

There is a way to get our bearings. When you're in a fog, get a compass. I have one—and you do too. We got our compass the day we decided to be healers. Our compass is a question, and it will point us true north: How will it help the patient?

This patient has a name. It is "Isaiah." He once lived. He was my patient. I dedicate this lecture to him.

You will soon learn a lovely lesson about doctoring; I guarantee it. You will learn that in a professional life that will fly by fast and hard, a hectic life in which thousands of people will honor you by bringing to you their pain and confusion, a few of them will stand out. For reasons you will not control and may never understand, a few will hug your heart, and they will become for you touch points—signposts—like that big boulder on that favorite hike that, when you spot it, tells you exactly where you are. If you allow it—and you should allow it—these patients will enter your soul, and you will, in a way entirely right and proper, love them. These people will be your teachers.

Isaiah taught me. He was fifteen when I met him. It was 1984, and I was the officer of the day—the duty doctor in my pediatric practice at the old Harvard Community Health Plan. My nurse practitioner partner pointed to an exam room. "You better get in there," she said. "That kid is in pain."

He was in pain. Isaiah was a tough-looking, inner-city kid. I would have crossed the street to avoid meeting him alone on a Roxbury corner at night. I'm not proud of that fact, but I admit it. But here on my examining table he was writhing, sweating in pain. He was yelling obscenities at the air, and, when I tried to examine him, he yelled them at me. "Don't you f——g touch me! Do something!"

I didn't figure out what was going on that afternoon. Nothing made sense. I diagnosed, illogically, a back sprain, and I sent him home on analgesics. Then, that evening, the report came: an urgent call from the lab. Isaiah didn't have a back sprain; he had acute lymphoblastic leukemia—ALL. And we didn't have his phone number.

The police helped track him down that night, to a lonely three-decker, third floor, a solitary house in a weedy lot on Sheldon Street in the heart of Roxbury. Isaiah lived there with his mother, brothers, and his mother's foster children.

What followed was the best of care . . . the glory of biomedical science came to Isaiah's service. Chemotherapy started, and he went predictably into remission. But we knew that ALL in a black teenager behaves badly. Unlike in younger kids, cure was unlikely. He would go into remission for a while, but the cancer would come back and it would kill him. Three years later, he relapsed.

I drove to his apartment one evening in 1987 and sat with Isaiah and his graceful, dignified mother around a table with a plastic, red-checkered tablecloth and explained the only option we knew for possible cure: a bone marrow transplant, not when he felt sick, but now, at the first sign of relapse, when he was still feeling fine. He was feeling fine, and I was there to propose treatment that might kill him.

They didn't hesitate. Isaiah wanted to live. He got his transplant, from his brother. His course was stormy, admission after admission followed, then chronic complications of his transplant—diabetes and asthma. His Children's Hospital medical record that year took up five four-inch-thick volumes. But he got through. Isaiah was cured.

We became very close, Isaiah and I, through this time and for years after—long conversations about his life, his hopes, his worries. He always asked me about my kids. And his mother, close, as well. An angel—a tough angel raised by her sharecropper grandfather on a North Carolina farm, who read Isaiah the riot act when she had to and who fiercely protected him—and who, during the darkest times of his course, continued to tend her ten foster children as well as her own.

I came to know Isaiah well, but it wouldn't be quite right to call us friends—our worlds were too far apart—different galaxies. But my respect and affection for Isaiah grew and grew. His courage. His insight. His generosity.

But there is more to tell.

Isaiah smoked his first dope at age five. He got his first gun before ten, and, by twelve, he had committed his first armed robbery; he was on crack at fourteen. Even on chemotherapy, he was in and out of police custody. For months after his transplant he tricked me into extra prescriptions for narcotics, which he hoarded and probably sold. Two of his five brothers were in jail—one for murder; and, two years into Isaiah's treatment, a third brother was shot dead—a gun blast through the front door—in a drug dispute.

Isaiah didn't finish school, and he had no idea of what to do for legitimate work. He lost job after job for not showing up or being careless. His world was the street corner, and his horizon was only one day away. He saw no way out. He hated it, but he saw no way out. He once told me that he thought his leukemia was a blessing, because at least while he was in the hospital, he couldn't be on the streets.

And Isaiah died. One night, eighteen years after his leukemia was cured, at thirty-seven years of age, they found him on a street corner, breathing but brain-dead from a prolonged convulsion from uncontrolled diabetes and even more uncontrolled despair.

Isaiah tried to phone me just before that fatal convulsion. He had my home number, and I still have the slip of paper on which my daughter wrote, "Isaiah called. Please call him back." I never did. He would have said, "Hi, Dr. Berwick. It's Isaiah. I'm really sick. I can't take it. I don't know what to do. Please help me." Because that is what he often said.

Isaiah spent the last two years of his life in a vegetative state in a nursing home where I sometimes visited him. At his funeral, his family asked me to speak, and I could think of nothing to talk about except his courage.

Isaiah, my patient. Cured of leukemia. Killed by hopelessness.

I bring Isaiah today as my witness to two duties; you have both. It's where your compass points.

First, you will cure his leukemia. You will bring the benefits of biomedical science to him, no less than to anyone else. Isaiah's poverty, his race, his troubled lifeline—not one of these facts or any other fact should stand in the way of his right to care—his human right to care. Let the Supreme Court have its day. Let the erratics and vicissitudes of politics play out their careless games. No matter. Health care is a human right; it must be made so in our nation; and it is your duty to make it so. Therefore, for your patients, you will go to the mat, and you will not lose your way. You are a physician, and you have a compass, and it points true north to what the patient needs. You will put the patient first.

But that is not enough. Isaiah's life and death testify to a further duty, one more subtle, but no less important. Maybe this second is not a duty that you meant to embrace; you may not welcome it. It is to cure, not only the killer leukemia; it is to cure the killer injustice.

Antoine de Saint-Exupéry wrote, "To become a man is to be responsible; to be ashamed of miseries that you did not cause." I say this: to profess to be a healer, that is, to take the oath you take today, is to be responsible; to be ashamed of miseries that you did not cause. That is a heavy burden, and you did not ask for it. But look at the facts.

In our nation—in our great and wealthy nation—the wages of poverty are enormous. The proportion of our people living below the official poverty line has grown from its low point of 11 percent in 1973 to more than 15 percent today; among children, it is 22 percent: 16.4 million; among black Americans, it is 27 percent. In 2010, more than forty-six million Americans were living in poverty; twenty million, in extreme poverty—incomes below $11,000 per year for a family of four. One million American children are homeless. More people are poor in the United States today than at any other time in our nation's history; 1.5 million American households, with 2.8 million children, live here on less than $2 per person per day. And fifty million more Americans live between the poverty line and just 50 percent above it—the near-poor, for whom, in the words of the Urban Institute, "The loss of a job, a cut in work hours, a serious health problem, or a rise in housing costs can quickly push them into greater debt, bankruptcy's brink, or even homelessness." For the undocumented immigrants within our borders, it's even worse.

For all of these people, our nation's commitment to the social safety net—the portion of our policy and national investment that reaches help to the disadvantaged—is life's blood. And today that net is fraying—badly. In 2010, twenty states eliminated optional Medicaid benefits or decreased coverage. State social services block grants and food stamps are under the gun. Enrollment in the TANF program—Temporary Assistance to Needy Families—has lagged far behind the need. Let me be clear: the will to eradicate poverty in the United States is wavering—it is in serious jeopardy.

In the great entrance hall of the building where I worked at CMS—the Hubert Humphrey Building, headquarters of the Department of Health and Human Services—are chiseled in massive letters the words of the late Senator Humphrey at the dedication of the building in his name. He said, "The moral test of government is how it treats those who are in the dawn of life, the children; those who are in the twilight of life, the aged; and those in the shadows of life, the sick, the needy and the handicapped."

This is also, I believe, the moral test of professions. Those among us in the shadows—they do not speak, not loudly. They do not often vote. They do not contribute to political campaigns or PACs. They employ no lobbyists. They write no op-eds. We pass by their coin cups outstretched, as if invisible, on the corner as we head for Starbucks; and Congress may pass them by too, because they don't vote, and, hey, campaigns cost money. And if those in power do not choose of their own free will to speak for them, the silence descends.

Isaiah was born into the shadows of life. Leukemia could not overtake him, but the shadows could, and they did.

I am not blind to Isaiah's responsibilities; nor was he. He was embarrassed by his failures; he fought against his addictions, his disorganization, and his temptations. He tried. I know that he tried. To say that the cards were stacked against him is too glib; others might have been able to play his hand better. I know that; and he knew that.

But to ignore Isaiah's condition not of his choosing, the harvest of racism, the frailty of the safety net, the vulnerability of the poor, is simply wrong. His survival depended not just on proper chemotherapy, but, equally, on a compassionate society.

I am not sure when the moral test was put on hold; when it became negotiable; when our nation in its political discourse decided that it was uncool to make its ethics explicit and its moral commitments clear—to the people in the dawn, the twilight, and the shadows. But those commitments have never in my lifetime been both so vulnerable and so important.

You are not confused; the world is. You need not forget your purpose, even if the world does. Leaders are not leaders who permit pragmatics to quench purpose. Your purpose is to heal, and what needs to be healed is more than Isaiah's bone marrow; it is our moral marrow—that of a nation founded on our common humanity. My brother, a retired schoolteacher, tells me that he always gets goose bumps when he reads this phrase: "We, the people . . ." We—you, and me, and Isaiah—inclusive.

It is time to recover and celebrate a moral vocabulary in our nation—one that speaks without apology or hesitation of the right to health care—the human right—and, without apology or hesitation, of the absolute unacceptability of the vestiges of racism, the violence of poverty, and blindness to the needs of the least powerful among us.

Now you don your white coats, and you enter a career of privilege. Society gives you rights and license it gives to no one else, in return for which you promise to put the interests of those for whom you care ahead of your own. That promise and that obligation give you voice in public discourse simply because of the oath you have sworn. Use that voice. If you do not speak, who will?

If Isaiah needs a bone marrow transplant, then, by the oath you swear, you will get it for him. But Isaiah needs more. He needs the compassion of a nation, the generosity of a commonwealth. He needs justice. He needs a nation to recall that, no matter what the polls say, and no matter what happens to be temporarily convenient at a time of political combat and economic stress, that the moral test transcends convenience. Isaiah, in his legions, needs those in power—you—to say to others in power that a nation that fails to attend to the needs of those less fortunate among us risks its soul. That is your duty, too.

This is my message from Isaiah's life and from his death. Be worried, but do not for one moment be confused. You are healers, every one, healers ashamed of miseries you did not cause. And your voice—every one—can be loud, and forceful, and confident, and your voice will be trusted. In his honor—in Isaiah's honor—please, use it.

Chapter 16

AND WE SAID, "NO"

COMMENTARY

Patricia A. Gabow

FOR MORE THAN two decades, Don Berwick has urged all of us in health care to aim to achieve greater safety, better quality, more responsible stewardship, and a clearer focus on the patient, the family, and the population. In his 2012 National Forum keynote address, he celebrates that "we have come a long way, baby," in these health care domains. But, Dr. Berwick is not a man to stop partway along a path to a better American health care system.

In this speech, Don presents his greatest challenge yet—not just to those of us in health care, but to all Americans, especially our leaders. He is asking us to see the truth, to articulate the truth, and to work to guarantee that what is true is also what is right and good. Achieving this clarity of thinking and action will be a long and difficult journey because there are many threatening and sometimes scary obstacles on this path. Dr. Berwick names "eleven hard-to-mention topics": the obstacles that we must address together to meet the challenge he has placed before us.

I want to focus on one of these "unmentionables" that affects many of the other ten: profit. One of my Italian grandfather's old sayings immediately comes to mind: "Too much is like not enough." Clearly, making some profit is acceptable, even desirable and needed, but the "hard-to-mention" part, Don says, is this: "We have come to accept the unbridled pursuit of revenue as okay even when it's a destructive game." He provides us with four examples of drugs whose development, marketing, and use reflect a zeal for unbridled profitability. Lest we think that excessive profit is the sole domain of the pharmaceutical industry, read Steven Brill's *Time* magazine article, "Bitter Pill: Why Medical Bills Are Killing Us." Brill documents hospital administrators with compensation over a million dollars; hospital profits of 26 percent; a device maker stockholders' "compounded annual return of 14.95 percent from 1990 to 2010"; and Washington health care lobbying expenditures of $5.36 billion since 1998.

American health care is a $2.8 trillion-per-year industry. If American health care were a country, it would have the fifth largest GDP in the world. That stack of $2.8 trillion is the biggest obstacle on the road, blocking us from achieving Dr. Berwick's challenge to "name the truth." The drive not just to keep the stack of health care dollars from decreasing, but to make it grow even bigger, blocks necessary and important changes at all the levels of health care and in our political system.

This obstacle has built up over decades. In 1961, President Dwight D. Eisenhower warned of the dangers of America's growing military-industrial complex in his farewell address to the nation: "This conjunction of immense military establishment and large arms industry is new in the American experience. The total influence—economic, political, even spiritual—is felt in every city, every state house, every office of the federal government. . . . In the councils of government we must guard against the acquisition of unwarranted influence, whether sought or unsought, by the military industrial complex."

It does not take much imagination to see the clear and unmistakable parallel to the similarly developing "medical-industrial complex" as city, state, and federal governments have paid the private sector to deliver health care just as it utilized private industry to develop our military might. In 1971, Ehrenreich and Ehrenreich introduced the concept of the medical-industrial complex as the industry "composed of multibillion dollar congeries of enterprises including doctors, hospitals, nursing homes, insurance companies, drug manufacturers, hospital supply and equipment companies, real estate and construction businesses, health system consulting and accounting firms and banks"—quite a list—and we could now add even more! They concluded that "an important (if not primary) function of the health care system in the United States is business (that is, to make profit)." The ensuing thirty years have taken us to an even more sobering reality.

In 1980, one of my mentors, Dr. Arnold Relman, was the first physician to call out this "medical-industrial complex." For three decades, he has continued to point out its insidious erosion of the health care profession and the health care system.

So, how do we meet Dr. Berwick's challenge? How do we make what is true about our health care system be what is right? If only we knew the answer. What we do know is that we must start naming the issue. A former Colorado governor, Richard Lamm, once said that problem solving has four phases: "No talk, no do; talk, no do; talk, do; and no talk, do." At the beginning of the cycle, we don't even name the problem; then we start to talk about it—put it on the table, give it a name. This is the beginning of problem solving. Then, we're talking and we're taking action to solve the problem. Finally, we have no need to discuss it anymore, we just do it.

Two decades ago, Dr. Berwick got us talking and then acting on the issues of quality, safety, and focus on the patient, family, and community. Now, he is exhorting us to start talking about the "eleven hard-to-mention" issues facing health care today. Just as we seized the previous challenges, let us all seize this challenge. It is our duty, not just for the patients; it is our duty to ourselves, to our children, and to the country.

FURTHER READING

Brill S. Bitter pill: Why medical bills are killing us. *Time*. February 26, 2013.

Ehrenreich B, Ehrenreich J, Health/PAC. *The American Health Empire: Power, Profits, and Politics*. New York: Vintage Books; 1971.

Eisenhower DD. Farewell address, January 17, 1961. Box 38
    Speech Series, Papers of Dwight D. Eisenhower as President
    1953–1961. Eisenhower Library: National Archives and
    Record Administration.

Estes CL, Harrington C, Pellow DN. Medical-industrial complex
    1818–1832. In: Borgatta E, Montgomery R (eds.).
    Encyclopedia of Sociology, 2nd edition. Framington Hills,
    MI: Gale Group; 2000.

Relman AS. The new medical-industrial complex. *N Engl J Med.*
    1980;303:963–970.

AND WE SAID, "NO"

PLENARY ADDRESS
INSTITUTE FOR HEALTHCARE IMPROVEMENT
24TH ANNUAL NATIONAL FORUM ON QUALITY
IMPROVEMENT IN HEALTH CARE
ORLANDO, FLORIDA, DECEMBER 12, 2012

IT'S A TRADITION in my Forum speeches for me to talk about my family. You met Nathaniel, my first grandson, just after he was born, when I spoke at the Forum in 2009, just before I went to Washington. In 2010, he was walking, and he knew about a hundred words. Like most two-year-olds, he could name four body parts, count to five, and stack six blocks.

He's three years old now. What a difference! This summer, during the Red Sox debacle, he was on the swings at the playground, and didn't want to leave. My daughter's fiancé, Joey, tried to help. Joey said, "Come on, the Red Sox are on TV; we can see Big Papi play." (Big Papi is the Red Sox designated hitter, David Ortiz.) Nathaniel's answer (and remember that he couldn't say one single sentence one year ago) was, "No, we can't see Big Papi; Big Papi's on the DL." (The disabled list.)

My wife was driving with Nathaniel last month and pulled into a gas station. This little guy, who couldn't put on his own shoes a year ago, looked out the window at the pump island, and asked, "What the heck is a fire extinguisher doing at a gas station?"

Now, I am not saying that Nathaniel is a genius. Well, he *is* a genius, but that's not the *point* of my story. What I am saying is, "Wow! Where did *that* come from?" Child development sneaks up on you like bread rising in the oven. That's one of the great joys of being a pediatrician—to see that.

That's one of the great joys of watching the health care improvement movement, too. Over and over again, I think, "Wow! Where did *that* come from?"

How far have we come? Well, I remember meeting with a group of orthopedists thirty years ago, maybe in 1985 or so, and they were forming a quality assurance committee. I said, "Why don't you call it a quality *improvement* committee?" "We can't do that," said one of the docs. "If we did that people might think we were doing something wrong now." I don't think that would happen today.

In 1983, I was collecting patient satisfaction data at the Harvard Community Heath Plan, where I worked, and I presented it to an internal medicine group meeting there. One of the doctors—Carol—a friend of mine—stood up in the back of the room, crumpled her feedback report into a ball, threw it at me, and walked out of the room. Today, I don't think she would.

Thirty years ago, we didn't know patient safety was a problem. Health care infections simply came with the territory. "Patient-centered care" meant a focus group or two. And most doctors laughed at checklists—"cookbook medicine."

That was then. This is now. We have come a long way, baby! Through 2012, I have been traveling all over the United States and to other countries, discovering—rediscovering—how much progress we've made.

- I have found the Associates in Process Improvement *Model for Improvement* papering the walls in small clinics in rural Oregon and in large hospitals in Auckland, New Zealand.
- I have seen the Central Line Bundle sweep across America, reducing bacteremia cases by tens of thousands.
- I saw Drs. Joe Harbison and Peter Kelly in Dublin use PDSA cycles with nurse practitioners to take stroke thrombolysis rates in Ireland from 2.4 percent in 2007 to a world-leading 9.5 percent.

- Dr. Ken McDonald and the irrepressible David Vaughn in Ireland, too, have helped take CHF three-month readmission rates in eight acute hospitals down to 6.9 percent, compared with the international best practice rate of 12 to 15 percent.

- I met Dr. David Ross, an ER physician in Denver, who is figuring out how to redirect EMT services to a new mission: keeping patients at home instead of automatically transporting them to hospitals.

- I have seen entire nations—New Zealand, Scotland, Denmark, Ireland, Singapore, Colombia—embrace patient safety and system improvement as public policy and national strategy.

- Our own country, in January 2011, approved a National Quality Strategy with John Whittington's and Tom Nolan's Triple Aim as its core.

- Best of all, I have seen the young people rise. The IHI Open School now has over 116,000 participating students in 550 Chapters in 58 countries. If you have met with them, as I have, then you don't just have hope for the future; you have certainty. Nothing is going to stop them.

But, we are not done. We are by no means done. In fact, from the viewpoint of scale—getting the changes everywhere that our reeling economies, our angry payers, and our fretful politicians need—we are miles from home. And, so, as I have marveled this year at the progress, I have also been asking myself, "Why not? What's in the way?"

I have come to a difficult conclusion. I think that we're scared of the truth. The next curve of change crosses some veiled and scary landscape.

My friend Scott Weingarten, the CEO of Zynx, which helps support evidence-based care, gave me a metaphor for what we face: the Choluteca Bridge.

The Choluteca River Bridge is in Honduras, Central America. It was built for strength in 1938. It proved its strength in 1995, when Hurricane Mitch came to Honduras. Mitch was a killer hurricane. It killed people and it also killed bridges—150 Honduran bridges fell during Hurricane Mitch, but not the Choluteca Bridge. It survived: strong, proud, as designed. Just one problem, though. The river moved. The Choluteca Bridge is still strong, but it's useless. It *was* in the right place, but *now*, it's in the *wrong* one.

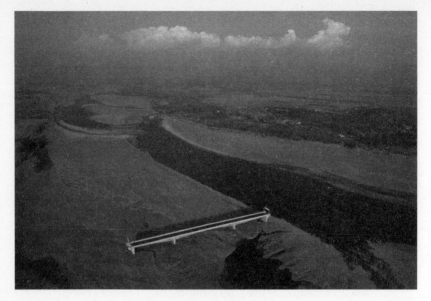

But, the River Moved . . .
Used with permission. © Vincent J. Musi, "The Bridge to Nowhere."

This, my friends, is American health care. Well—not totally so. After all, a river still runs under the system we built—the one we built for biotechnology, audacity, and miracles. We still need intensive care units and surgery suites and organ transplants and complex cancer care. Children died when I was in training who would have lived today—their hearts repaired, their leukemia cured. Let me pay homage to Dr. Joseph Murray, who died last month, the gracious, courageous Nobel Prize–winning surgeon who did the first renal transplant.

Bravo, miracles! We want them; and, with luck, we'll have more and more of them. But, we need new bridges . . . the bridges to prevention, to thriving despite chronic illness, to care in communities, and to health, itself. This talk is about what it's going to take to build them. And it's a scary talk.

Politics isn't helping right now: polarized, contentious. Political discourse does not yet know what we in the improvement world hold and share as central: customer focus; joy in work; that all improvement is change, though not all change is improvement; how to learn by testing changes. Far too few political leaders really understand that better quality is the best route to lower cost. We, in improvement, might even be excited that there is a new river to cross. Politics isn't.

So, instead, we get sound-bite grenades and thoughtless incivility, just when we most badly need tolerance for complexity—respectful dialogue even when we disagree—*especially* when we disagree. That is sad. In time, it will pass. Our nations are strong and our people are good, and government will come again to reflect that strength and goodness. But, meanwhile, there is too much silence about problems that we have to talk about if we are to make progress.

We and our leaders have been taught this silence. These problems become, like Voldemort, "he who shall not be named." "Shhh," we say, "we better not go there; people might think we are doing something wrong now. People like us."

That won't work. About ten years ago, we asked Gloria Steinem to speak at the National Forum to help us form the movement that became the IHI 100,000 Lives Campaign. She told us that one of the essential steps in mobilization is to give the problem a name. We could not fight date rape, she told us, until we created the name "date rape."

Europeans more than Americans use the term "civil society," and I think those words point exactly to daylight. *Civil* means nongovernmental, decorous, respectful, public, courteous. And *society* is a word for civilized interactions and dignified association.

What politics has temporarily made unspoken and hidden—the third rails in public debate—become an urgent agenda for civil society.

That's us. We *here* are civil society. We have a job to do: moving the bridge to the river. Bickering soloists or warring tribes can't do that. All of us—together—can.

So, follow me, please. And don't be afraid, even if it gets a little dark out there. We're going to name things.

Nathaniel, by the way, can teach us a thing or two about fear. At age three, he has recently discovered monsters. Bedtime can't happen until we (and I do mean "we") have checked the walls, the closets, and under the bed to make sure that the coast is clear. So far, no monsters. I'll keep you posted.

Let's check under *our* bed. I'll name eleven hard-to-mention topics. Each needs the best minds and the most creative expeditions, but almost all of them are more or less off-limits in political conversation. But, not for us. They come in four categories: (1) using knowledge; (2) addressing waste; (3) setting priorities; and (a singleton) (4) managing the transition.

First, the uses of knowledge.

1. *Confidence in Science.* A triumph, albeit incomplete, of twentieth-century health care was to decide to connect medical decisions to

science; to treat patients according to facts, not myths or habits. It's incomplete because we don't yet always do that—move knowledge from bench to bed—and partly because we have allowed senseless, unscientific variation to masquerade as autonomy. The result is a confused public. And now, it's a suspicious public. It is made suspicious by exploitive accusations that scientific thought is elitist, and that appealing to science is an excuse to take advantage of individuals—a way to deny people what they need. When we say, "science" and "evidence-based medicine," a lot of the public hears "rationing" and even "eugenics." That's just wrong, of course. It is exactly science that can best protect us from rationing, by allowing us to distinguish waste from help.

What can you do? Insist on care that is based on science, but—and this is very important—employ scientific thinking at the individual patient level. Use PDSA cycles to craft and adjust care for each individual patient, rather than using blunt, population-based results that do not take adequate account of individual variation. I'll talk more about that in minute.

2. *Using Global Brains.* When I went to D.C., I got intensive drilling to get ready for congressional hearings. I spent hours and hours with so-called murder boards, play-acting panels throwing questions at me that a senator might ask. My teachers gave me some rules as general guides, and the first rule they taught me was this: "Never mention another country." If I said, "Toyota," they suggested I say, "Ford."

Not thinking globally hurts us. Okay, so Americans *are* exceptional. So are Swedes, and Basques, and Oregonians, and Londoners. We *all* differ, sometimes gloriously, in heritage, talents, and resources. Everyone is exceptional. Being different isn't a bad thing. What's bad is to miss the chance to *learn* from our differences. Think of our differences as vast natural experiments—and they can teach us tons. Penicillin discovered in Paddington cures strep in Peoria, for Pete's sake.

This is for me, of course, personal, both because I have learned so much from colleagues all over the world, and because demagogues exploited the simple fact that I had praised elements of the British National Health Service to obstruct my confirmation as CMS administrator.

America suffers—patients suffer—if we close our eyes to what we can learn from anyone, anywhere. Using national exceptionalism as an excuse to blindfold ourselves makes no sense.

What can you do? Would the international—non-US—participants stand? Look at the abundance. Stop each other in the halls. Ask each other how you solve your problems. How do you use nurses in the community? How do you care for the frail elderly? How do you get so many young people interested in primary care? Make your brain a global brain.

3. *Learning in Large Systems.* If you want to improve health care, you are going to have to engage a messy world. You're not in a laboratory; you're in life. Normal experimentalist approaches to learning will not work. But, mostly, evaluation remains tethered to designs that are weak for learning. As what you're trying to change gets larger or more complex, you'd better adjust from evaluation to continual learning. And "evaluation" and "learning" are not the same task epistemologically. Try telling your spouse that you are "evaluating" your marriage, and see what happens. Actually, I suggest that you don't. But, you could ask, "What could I try tomorrow that would make our marriage even better?" And then, try it.

This confusion is strongly reflected in federal policy in the Congressional Budget Office's scoring rules for legislation and in decision making in the Office of Management and Budget, for example. It slows progress, it limits risk taking, and it discards lessons from the real world. A modern corporation that used CBO scoring rules to decide on the investments it makes in innovation would wither, overtaken by those who embrace discovery and understand prediction.

This has been a chronic battle over the epistemology of improvement, and it is time to end it. The best image I know of the problem is this from Lloyd Provost. From a still and peaceful pond, we can draw a sample of water, test it, and learn a lot about the whole pond. That's classical inference. But the world of care—the real world about which we wish to learn—is one not of still waters. It's rushing rivers. Sample once from the river, and you don't learn much about the future—the next sample. Learning in rushing waters of change is an exercise in prediction, not census taking, and the methods of learning that work in the torrent are different. Yet the stewards of scientific inquiry—our academicians and journal editorial boards—have neither sufficiently developed nor widely accepted new investigatory approaches. It is high time that they do so.

What can you do? Learn improvement science. Use control charts and study special causes. Use narratives from patients and families to start your learning journey.

The second category has to do with reducing waste.

4. *Naming the Excess.* America spends more on health care than it needs to—much more. A fifth grader would realize that if she simply glanced at the relationships between per capita spending among nations and national health status and care outcomes. And yet, it is far easier to sell the public on the claim that we need more . . . *fill in the blank* . . . than less. I think these claims are often good-hearted—you do need more if the chassis is broken. But it has become nearly impossible to claim that enough is enough, in the face of public fears of rationing, even though that's true.

This particular monster, the dimensions of excess, may be the scariest one under the bed. Let me show you how scary it can be. Dr. Bernard Lown, one of the most distinguished cardiologists in the world, helped invent the modern defibrillator, first worked out the relationships between digitalis and potassium, and won the Nobel Peace Prize in 1985 as the cofounder of International Physicians for the Prevention of Nuclear War. He is not a couch potato.

For years, Dr. Lown has studied overuse of coronary revascularization procedures—stents and CABG surgery. He has concluded, and he's written extensively about the evidence, that half or more of the revascularization procedures performed today for stable coronary disease in the United States are unnecessary. Half. They do not relieve symptoms any better than proper medical management does, nor do they lengthen life or prevent further heart attacks. Dr. Lown's belief, and the practice within the Lown Cardiovascular Group, which he founded, rests on medical management of symptoms, with at least as much success as if the same patients had been managed invasively. The Lown Institute has the data, and, by the way, they have never had a malpractice suit for the conservative approach to coronary disease.

I have spent time lately with Dr. Lown and his colleague, Vikas Sainy, and I find them convincing. And, though theirs is a minority view, they are by no means alone in it. But, I am not a cardiologist, and I am not presenting Lown's views to convince you of them. Rather, I simply want to raise a question: What if he were right?

Better check under the bed. Over six hundred thousand stents are placed in coronary arteries in the United States each year, and five hundred thousand CABG operations are done. Most of these patients have stable coronary disease. Just imagine for a minute what it would mean if Dr. Lown were right. All those angiography suites; all those gleaming ORs; all those proud and technically brilliant interventional cardiologists—what happens to them? What happens to the business models of the heart hospitals and the stent vendors? And so, when the evidence accumulates that what we do a lot of doesn't help nearly as much as we thought, it's scary to ask and easier not to.

And yet, we do see courage. With the brilliant leadership of the American Board of Internal Medicine Foundation in its "Choosing Wisely" Campaign, Shannon Brownlee and the New America Foundation, and a new effort spearheaded by Dr. Saini, who is president of the Lown Institute, our nation is taking a much closer look at overtreatment. But, beware; it takes courage to name and address the large proportion of American health care that simply does not help. The forces to turn the inquiry aside will be massive.

Here is the good news. Imagine all the good we could do with what we could harvest from the reduction of excess. It would put universal coverage much more within reach. It would allow us to put programs and people where the need really is. We could build the new bridge.

5. *Profit.* We have come too much to accept the unbridled pursuit of revenue as okay even when it's a destructive game. The American health care marketplace is an odd combination of, on the one hand, generative, energizing entrepreneurship and proper competition and, on the other hand, calculating, cynical greed. We lack sufficient methods in public policy and private notice to tell the difference and to act on it. Prosecuting outright fraud and corruption is not the same as interdicting greed whose army is lawyers, but the latter can be as destructive as real crime; it undermines both the public treasury and the public trust. Let me tell you four stories:

• *Makena:* This is a simple, cheap chemical—basically 17-hydroxy progesterone—which is effective in interrupting premature labor, which reduces low birth weight among babies. A course of treatment with the generic compound costs about $15 per dose, or $300. But a drug company, KV Pharmaceutical, took advantage of a loophole in the orphan drug law to patent 17-hydroxy progesterone as "Makena," at

$25,000 per course of treatment. Fifty percent of the births in this country are in Medicaid, and the threat and costs of low birth weight are concentrated in families with economic and social disadvantage. To avoid pushback from the powerful, KV Pharmaceutical heavily discounted Makena to patients with private insurance; but it applied its shelf price, $25,000, to Medicaid patients. The cost to Medicaid: over $1 billion per year. When the FDA issued guidance that said it would not enforce restriction on compounding pharmacies providing the generic drug at cost, KV Pharmaceutical sued and lost in federal court.

- *Lucentis:* A powerful drug company, Genentech, makes the anti-tumor drug, Avastin (bevacizumab), which is widely used. Genentech also produces a very closely related chemical for intraocular injection use against wet macular degeneration, which affects mainly the Medicare population, under the brand name, Lucentis (ranibuzimab). The two drugs have been shown in randomized trials to be equally effective. For the equivalent amount of the chemical—the amount used for one intraocular injection—Avastin costs $50 per dose and Lucentis costs $2,000. Some ophthalmologists, trying to keep costs down for patients, whose copayment is substantial, buy Avastin and dilute it in their offices. This is, by the way, against the economic interests of the doctors, who get paid 6 percent of the costs of the Medicare Part B drugs they use. Other ophthalmologists just use Lucentis. The cost to Medicare of Lucentis versus Avastin is $1.4 billion per year, and 20 percent of that cost is born by beneficiaries themselves. Lucentis costs beneficiaries $400 per dose; Avastin costs $11. Genentech could make Avastin available in intraocular concentrations and leave the clinical choice to ophthalmologists. But, they don't. There is too much money in Lucentis.

- *Colcrys:* Colchicine has been used for the treatment of gout for three thousand years. Technically, though, it was a so-called unapproved drug under FDA rules until it was formally evaluated in 2009 in a trial by a company called URL Pharma, which the FDA then gave exclusive rights to: rights to a three-thousand-year-old drug costing 9 cents a pill until then. URL boosted the price fifty-fold to $4.85 a pill, or up to $3,600 a year for patients previously paying one-fiftieth of that price. In 2007, the total Medicaid payment for colchicine was about

$1 million a year. For Colcrys—the same drug—it's over $50 million a year.

- *Erythropoetin and Bundled Payment:* The very first Medicare bundled payment is for hemodialysis. I actually call it a "bundlet," because it just covers time, professional fees, and drugs for one dialysis session. When the baseline was set for the bundled payment, the cost of erythrocyte stimulating factor (EPO) was included, because the standard of care at that moment encouraged doctors to drive patients' hemoglobin levels above 10 grams per deciliter. In fact, under the Affordable Care Act, the quality incentive bonus for dialysis care included target hemoglobin levels.

  But, while this was all playing out, the science changed. It became clearer that high hemoglobin levels were associated with *worse* outcomes for patients with chronic renal failure, and that there was insufficient scientific evidence for maintaining hemoglobin at any specific level. So, a revision of the quality incentive structure was issued while I was administrator, and the use of EPO began to fall. But this was *after* the benchmark for the dialysis bundle was set with EPO costs *in* the benchmark. The effect was a major windfall to dialysis providers, who, in essence, kept receiving payment for the former rates of use of a drug whose use should and did decrease; the windfall approached a half-billion dollars in the first half of 2011. The dialysis industry, of course, took the money.

Now, let me be clear. These companies are doing what makes sense to them; they are generally playing by the rules—nothing illegal. But, not everything legal is proper. It's the rules that are wrong: pricing rules, licensing rules, payment rules, and more. They leave too much room for behaviors that, even if legal, are cynical, harmful, and extremely costly.

Check under the bed. Monsters lurk when you try to change those rules, and civil society would have to give the politicians and legislators the courage to change.

What can you do? Where you work, you can act differently. You can aim for fairness; you can share your gains. And, as citizens, you can use your voice to tell those who work for you in government to draw solid lines between fair profit, which we can live with, and cynical greed, which we will not.

6. *Innovations That Do Not Help.* The password for the year—maybe for the decade—is "innovation." That's encouraging, because all improvement is change. On the other hand, not all

change is improvement, and not all innovations help. Indeed, at
this stage in health care, I have a feeling that many—maybe
most—of the changes in health care equipment, products, and
services that get labeled "innovations" may not help. I am not
saying that they have high, but positive, marginal cost-benefit
ratios; those pose a different problem of societal choice. I am
saying that they have *negative* marginal cost-benefit ratios: worse
care at higher cost. I spoke earlier this year at a major annual
clinical convention with six thousand participants. The organizers
toured me through the exhibit hall, and told me that there were
six thousand vendors there. I saw their wares, some in giant
trailers that had been driven into the exhibit hall and transformed
into house-sized displays—fiber optic this, robotic that, exotic
new ceramics, and disposable everything. I am sure that
somewhere in that acreage of innovations are a few miracles,
able to help patients, and definitely worth the money. But every
instinct I have whispers to me that most—maybe almost all of
what I saw—is not just not worth the money, but will add
complexity, risks, and downstream opportunity costs.

And yet, public policy can do nearly nothing about it. The statutory
authority in Medicare and Medicaid to demand evidence, inform clinicians, and tie it all to payment is weak or nonexistent. One important
counter-example, the Affordable Care Act provision that Medicare has
to cover any clinical preventive practices scored A or B by the US Preventive Services Task Force, has been attacked as government-run medical
care. With very few exceptions, neither the FDA nor CMS can consider
cost or comparative cost-effectiveness in any of its findings. The mechanisms for coverage decisions in Medicare are few and administratively
starved. And market forces have not shown the strength to distinguish
between helpful innovations and unhelpful ones.

You can be different. You can go back to science and learning, with
healthy skepticism about the newest gadget. Who, if anyone, really, does
it help, and under what conditions? You can master Lean thinking and
Lean production.

7. *Boundaries of Guilds.* Health care has proud professions, and
   they have strong guilds. I think these professions deserve our
   respect and our trust in their ethics and generosity. But, their
   guilds need to change. For example, they could not oppose, but
   support, new models of care—models like expanded roles for

nonphysicians, new power for patients and families, bold uses for telemedicine. Let me give you three quick examples:

a. The ECHO project in New Mexico, led by Dr. Sanjeev Arora, which is now achieving the same results for Hepatitis C cure in rural, primary care New Mexico via telemedicine as for patients who are referred to the University Medical Center

b. The AFHCAN Cart in Alaska, which is linking remote Alaska Native villages throughout Alaska telemetrically to consultative resources in Anchorage, providing nearly instant access and cutting travel for face-to-face visits by 70 percent

c. The DHAT program in Alaska, a program of the Alaska Native Tribal Health Consortium and the University of Washington, which is training young people—even high school graduates—in Alaska to provide primary dental care to remote villages without the need for a dentist

The legacy payment patterns, RBRVS payment, coding systems, and rules don't encourage changes like these. They make them harder. Especially the rules on scope of practice are way behind the times.

We need the help of the guilds, not their opposition. I spoke a few weeks ago to the annual meeting of a specialty society. The explicit theme of the meeting was advancing patient safety. But here is how they interpreted that goal: "Stop expanded roles for nurses." I do not agree. It's time to change.

So, help with the change. Instead of resisting the new roles and technologies, ask, with optimism, how to make them continually safer, more reliable, and more effective. Instead of saying, "No," ask, "How?"

The third category has to do with setting priorities in innovation.

8. *Defending the Poor.* In my Forum speech last year, I showed you the quotation from Senator Hubert Humphrey that is engraved in the wall of the Great Hall of the headquarters building of HHS—the Hubert Humphrey Building: "The moral test of government is how it treats those in the dawn of life, the children; those in the twilight of life, the aged; and those in the shadows of life, the sick, the needy and the handicapped." At the moment, that is a hard sell in the public arena. I am not exactly sure why, but I guess that polls suggest that defending the safety net doesn't get you a lot of votes. If you tune into the politics, you'd think at the moment that the moral test of

government is how it treats the middle class. Of course the middle class is important, and I totally agree with the agenda that that leads us to: jobs, infrastructure, tax restraint, and so on. But, I am losing sleep about Hubert Humphrey's moral test. We are at risk of failing it. The social safety net is vulnerable. The will to protect the poor needs constant reinforcement from civil society; government won't do it without that fuel. Voldemort, scat! Health care is a human right—period.

And, remember, you with global brains, our international colleagues are giving care at something like half of our US costs. How do they do that? If we understand that, how much more will we have available to ensure that everybody gets care?

9. *End-of-Life Care.* The cruel rhetoric about "death panels" has taken end-of-life care frankly off the political table, at just the time that an aging population and an entirely new profile of chronic illness demand the opposite. "Death panels," of course, are hogwash—pure figments of warped imagination, and of irresponsible leaders willing to frighten vulnerable people in the service of selfish political gain. Yet, the rules in Washington are clear: never officially mention care at the end of life, palliative care, or advance directives. That silence is tragic; and it has to stop. So, join The Conversation Project; study and replicate the success in La Crosse, Wisconsin; and speak up everywhere about the possibility of far, far better care in advanced illness and at the end of life.

10. *Authentic Prevention.* Of the three dimensions of the IHI Triple Aim—better care, better health, lower cost—the runt of the litter is better health. Those cathedrals of our time—hospitals—cure disease; they do not prevent it. And, of course, mostly they *cannot* prevent it, because they are nowhere near the changeable causes: behavioral choices, nutrition, inequity, injustice, pollution, and so on. Prevention has no cathedrals. The result is a massive misallocation of effort and resources; a Martian visitor would call it insane. Simply put, we have not built sufficient institutional structures for the prevention of disease.

I saw a thrilling counter-example in September on a visit to New Zealand, where the cabinet-level Commission for Children—yes, New Zealand has a cabinet-level officer just for kids—issued the plan for ending childhood poverty in New Zealand. The plan is comprehensive; it's about jobs, housing, health care, education, and infrastructure. It's about prevention in its fullest form and led from the top. If they stick with it, it will work. Meanwhile, in the United States the prevention funds established in the Affordable Care Act are under attack, and there are serious proposals to cut the CDC budget in half. What we need is the opposite: a groundbreaking, habit-breaking redesign of our nation's approach to the prevention of illness and the preservation of health. We have the rhetoric—a national prevention strategy exists. But now we'll need the will and the institutional forms to make it real.

And let me mention a fourth category of barrier, with just a single entry.

11. *Business Transition Models.* In my National Forum speech last year, I called attention to one of the finest innovations in American health care delivery that I have ever seen: the Nuka care system for Alaska Natives, led by the Southcentral Foundation in Anchorage, Alaska, which won the 2009 Malcolm Baldrige National Quality Award. You may recall that Nuka is a team-based, population-minded, prevention-oriented total care system built solidly on principles of total cooperation. The results are stunning. Nuka care has driven ED visits down by 50 percent, hospital bed days down by 53 percent, specialist visits by 65 percent, primary care visits by 20 percent, all while achieving excellent quality scores and the highest patient and staff satisfaction in their history. Results like that, at national scale, would totally solve the US health care problem without harming a single patient. But, a normal US hospital executive or specialist who saw these results wouldn't feel elated; she'd feel heartburn. The hospital CEO would be at risk of being fired by the board as revenues fell. The problem isn't the destination; it's the transition: stranded capital, a misaligned workforce, business cycle management, and public belief that confuses volume and technology with healing and solace. I think that US health care executives and boards are starting to get it, but few know how to navigate that transition, and it worries them. As a result, the adaptations of American hospitals to the new game are often *maladaptive.* Their foundations are revenue models and last-man-standing business models that cannot work for American communities in the years ahead.

Ladies and gentlemen, meet Voldemort. Eleven monsters; they'd like to scare us into silence.

Soon, Nathaniel will leave his monsters behind. So should we. The improvement movement can celebrate three decades of growing success now—case by case, process by process. Bravo! Now, some monsters ahead. "They roar their terrible roars, and gnash their terrible teeth; and roll their terrible eyes; and show their terrible claws."

That's from Maurice Sendak's *Where the Wild Things Are*. Nathaniel knows it nearly by heart. I do, too. We love the part where the monsters say to Max: "Oh, please don't go. We'll eat you up; we love you so." And Max says, "No!" That's our job. Us, too: "No."

Here is what we will do, loudly, constantly, and unafraid:

1. Reaffirm confidence in science as the basis for helping and cure.

2. Learn unapologetically, not just within nations, but among nations.

3. Learn to learn in complex systems, which defy classical experiments, but which nonetheless are rich with lessons.

4. Declare that overtreatment is widespread in care, and that we will stop it.

5. Neither engage in nor tolerate in silence profiteering that harms patients and degrades public trust.

6. Require that innovations show their worth before they spread.

7. Call upon and lead the professional guilds to embrace change. They need to welcome widening scopes of practice, and to participate whole-heartedly in the redesign of health care as a system.

8. Defend the poor, the children, and the aged. We will pass the moral test.

9. Improve—no, *revolutionize*—care approaching the end of life, to ensure human dignity, comfort, and the healing presence of loved ones and community.

10. Honor prevention not in rhetoric, but in fact.

11. Develop, test, share, and spread pragmatic models for health care organizations to make the transition from volume-based business models to integrated care directed at the Triple Aim.

This isn't small stuff. It brings the improvement movement—you—fully into contact with the politics and pressures of systemic change—not a place you or I thought we would be. But, I think we *need* to be there. The bridge to the future is not the bridge of the past.

Nathaniel stands at a threshold. Soon he will leave behind the monsters in his mind, who "roar their terrible roars and gnash their terrible teeth." But, leaving behind the beasts he imagines, he will, of course, come face to face with the orcs and ogres of the real world. If he chooses a life of service, as you have, his role and mission will be to pull their fangs. Ours—our orcs, our ogres—the misuse of knowledge, the wages of waste, the tragedy of priorities misplaced—have the power of the past on their side. It will take power to fight power, and courage to change course.

Jeff Selberg, IHI's chief operating officer, gave me a gift by telling me these words from Paul Tillich: "Love without power will never achieve justice, and power without love will never be just." Love—power—justice. Think about it, because those three now, welcome or not, have become our task.

INDEX

A

AAMC. *See* Association of American Medical Colleges

Abernathy, Ralph, 207

ABIM (American Board of Internal Medicine) Foundation, 166, 257

ACA. *See* Affordable Care Act

Acute lymphoblastic leukemia (ALL), 239

Acute myocardial infarction (AMI), 32–38, 224

ADE (adverse drug event), prevention of, 35, 224

Administrative Complexity, as form of waste, 218–219

Advanced Access model (Murray and Tantau), 19

Advocate Good Samaritan Hospital (Chicago area), 59

Affordable Care Act (ACA), 123, 137, 178, 206, 209, 214, 215, 259, 260, 263

AFHCAN Cart (Alaska), 261

Agency for Healthcare Research and Quality (AHRQ), 33, 74, 81, 82, 142

AHRQ. *See* Agency for Healthcare Research and Quality

Alanya, Turkey, 191, 192

Alaska Native Medical Center (Anchorage, Alaska), 6, 19, 22

Alaska Native Tribal Health Consortium, 261

Allegheny Hospital (Pittsburgh, Pennsylvania), 34

Allina Health (Minneapolis), 74

Altruism, 128–129, 170, 172, 175

American Academy of Family Physicians (AAFP), 196

American Board of Internal Medicine Foundation (ABIM), 257

American College of Cardiology (ACC), 59, 80; door-to-balloon program, 105

American Health Quality Association, 81

American Heart Association, 59, 80; "Get With the Guidelines" program, 81

American Hospital Association (AHA), 62, 79, 81, 105; National Hospital Survey (2005), 75

American Medical Association (AMA), 74, 105

American Nurses Association (ANA), 74, 105; National Database of Nursing Quality Indicators, 81

AMI. *See* Acute myocardial infarction

Anchorage, Alaska, 185

Annals of Internal Medicine (Fisher), 13

Aristotle, 155

Arora, Sanjeev, 261

Ascension Health, 40, 42, 44, 74, 78, 82

Asheville, North Carolina, 187–188

Associates in Process Improvement, 141, 250

RA399.A3 B48 2014
Promising care : how we can
rescue health care by
improving it